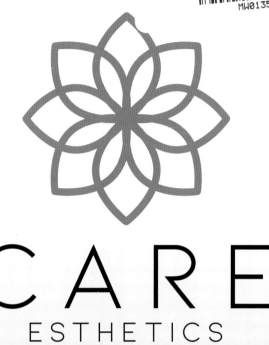

CARE
ESTHETICS

*A Healthy Way to Natural
Facial Rejuvenation*

Dedication

To the hundreds of doctors and CARE Esthetics providers who have contributed to the field of facial esthetics in a more natural approach. Your efforts continue to pave the way to a healthier attitude toward facial esthetics and regenerative medicine. Thank you for doing what's right.

Library of Congress Cataloging-in-Publication Data

Names: Miron, Richard J. (Richard John), 1983- editor.
Title: CARE Esthetics : a healthy way to natural facial rejuvenation / edited by Richard J. Miron.
Description: Chicago : Quintessence Publishing, 2021. | Includes bibliographical references and index. | Summary: "Explains the basics behind skin aging and facial rejuvenation before demonstrating the minimally invasive procedures available with PRF, lasers, and Botox/fillers as well as proper skin care to achieve natural facial rejuvenation instead of that plastic surgery look"-- Provided by publisher.
Identifiers: LCCN 2021045700 | ISBN 9781647241285 (paperback)
Subjects: LCSH: Face--Surgery. | Skin--Care and hygiene. | Dermatology.
Classification: LCC RD119.5.F33 C37 2021 | DDC 617.5/2059--dc23/eng/20211021
LC record available at https://lccn.loc.gov/2021045700

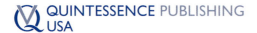

©2022 Quintessence Publishing Co, Inc

Quintessence Publishing Co, Inc
411 N Raddant Road
Batavia, IL 60510
www.quintpub.com

5 4 3 2 1

All rights reserved. This book or any part thereof may not be reproduced, stored in a retrieval system, or transmitted in any form or by any means, electronic, mechanical, photocopying, or otherwise, without prior written permission of the publisher.

Editor: Leah Huffman
Design: Sue Zubek
Production: Sue Robinson

Printed in the USA

Contents

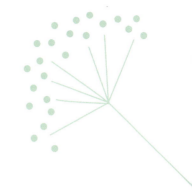

1. Introduction *1*
2. Aging and the Healing Process *7*
3. Foreign Body Reactions *27*
4. Why the Dentist? *39*
5. What Is Platelet-Rich Fibrin? *49*
6. Use of PRF in Facial Esthetics *57*
7. Lasers in Facial Esthetics *79*
8. Botox and Dermal Fillers *95*
9. Bio-Lift and Bio-CARE Protocols *111*
10. Cosmeceuticals and Skin Care *121*
11. The Future of Regenerative Medicine *141*
12. What to Expect with Treatment *149*

Chapter 1

Introduction

First, I'd like to start by introducing myself. I am one of the many CARE Esthetics providers in the country who has helped contribute to this book for the betterment of our patients. You may wonder: What exactly is CARE Esthetics?

CARE Esthetics stands for the **C**enter for **A**dvanced **R**ejuvenation and **E**sthetics and was established several years ago due to the growing patient demand for minimally invasive facial esthetic and regenerative procedures performed in the safest, most effective, and most natural way possible. We have become one of the largest facial esthetics groups in the world (Fig 1), which allows us to rapidly accumulate new information and knowledge as thousands of procedures are being performed throughout our many clinics across the United States. Just think about it: If each provider tries a new therapy 10 times in an organized group with 100 clinics, 1,000 cases would be performed using that unique new technology. As a single provider, I would only have access and experience from my 10 cases. But by joining CARE Esthetics and teaming up with like-minded clinicians, I can now learn from all 1,000 cases. Together we learn faster, share experiences faster, and ultimately deliver better therapies faster for the benefit of our patients.

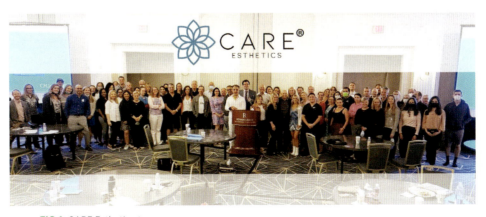

FIG 1 CARE Esthetics team.

At CARE Esthetics, our providers include medically trained professionals from many backgrounds by design. Some are daily clinical providers who have years of experience in the field. Some are clinical researchers based out of universities who have developed some of the technologies we use daily in clinical practice. Some are plastic surgeons with the ability to handle complications quickly. Some are technology center professionals treating patients for the very first time with new technologies in research-based facilities (with informed consent from our patients of course). Together, through our shared experiences, we aim to advance the field collectively with one goal in mind—**to treat our patients the best way possible, in the safest way possible, in the most natural way possible**. You can only learn through experience, and our combined team has thousands of years of experience in the field. We continuously remain fully dedicated to providing the healthiest and safest regenerative strategies in facial esthetics to patients like you, and this book was written as an educational tool to give you an up-to-date guide on such therapies.

Our team is always growing. Some of our clinical researchers have PhDs in molecular and cell biology, which means that not only do they practice facial esthetics with patients, but they also spend time in a research facility investigating new technologies to the cellular and molecular level. The basis of their work involves the study of implanted medical devices/biomaterials into host tissues and exactly how the body interacts with these newly introduced substances. These biomaterials run the gamut from liquid growth factors to titanium dental/orthopedic implants and screws to human/animal graft tissues originating in cadavers or animal byproducts. Each of these biomaterials causes a foreign body reaction when it enters the body, which is basically the body's immune system deciding whether it likes this newly introduced material or not. To complicate matters, everyone's body is different. What may be perfectly well suited for one person may cause an allergic reaction in another. That is why this book discusses many types of chemical biomaterials/synthetic additives utilized in facial esthetics—to provide you with as much knowledge as possible prior to deciding for yourself which therapy you'd like to pursue to achieve your own personal goals and objectives.

After all, the goal of this book is NOT to encourage you to select one therapy over another. **The goal of this book is to give you accurate, up-to-date information that you can understand to inform your**

decisions about what you would like to introduce into your own body. There are no right or wrong choices, and the belief of every CARE Esthetics provider is that YOU should make the decision based on as much up-to-date information and knowledge as possible. Which route, products, or therapies you decide to pursue is up to you. In fact, you might read this entire book and decide that no therapy is right for you. That's perfectly okay. Your body is yours, and you—not I—should be making decisions about what you put into it. Far too often I have witnessed patients entering into facial procedures without adequate knowledge regarding their reasoning or choices or the potential long-term benefits or side effects of such choices. This book was written to fill that gap of knowledge and empower our patients to feel confident in their decisions. Read as much or as little of this book as you'd like. Skip around or read through all of the chapters. The choice is entirely yours!

The field of facial esthetics is booming, and the demand for such procedures has never been greater. Let's be honest: It's no secret that we all want to look better, to live longer and healthier lives, and to feel as young as possible for as long as possible. Because of societal pressures to look our best, new technologies in this field are being developed rapidly, some with exciting new outcomes and others with too much hype and too little scientific merit. This makes the field extremely exciting but also a bit scary at the same time. As an esthetic clinician, it is my job to break down this hype in order to provide you with the absolute best therapies out there.

Because our group joins over 100 clinics, each treating thousands of patients yearly, collectively we gather massive amounts of clinical data that we can scientifically assess in terms of patient satisfaction and clinical improvement. We compare new therapeutic discoveries and trends and share new technologies from various conferences we attend within our CARE Esthetics community. Our ability to collaborate collectively has placed us among the best minimally invasive facial esthetics clinics in the world, and clinicians from across the globe have been traveling to the US to learn from our group.

Another advantage of our size is that we can invest in the absolute best high-end technology (Fig 2). Technology startup costs are often too high for smaller individual clinics, potentially limiting the services that can be offered at such centers. By joining our clinics under the CARE franchise, we all benefit from lower bulk pricing for technology, and we are all required to

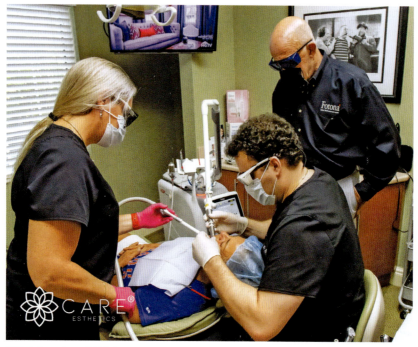

FIG 2 One of our CARE Esthetics providers using a Fotona laser system.

complete comprehensive training on these new therapies as well as yearly educational programs to stay active and up to date in the field. Safety is our top priority.

This book will cover existing therapies, including Botox, dermal fillers, laser therapy, platelet concentrates, PDO threads, and various surgical options. The book will always favor more natural and biocompatible regenerative strategies that utilize the body's own healing potential rather than the introduction of foreign substances or chemical fillers. But as highlighted throughout this book, the final choice is always and entirely yours. We are simply here to provide you with up-to-date information and answer any questions you may have. There are no right or wrong choices or bad questions. You can ask as many questions as you need to feel comfortable making your decision, and you can know that we stand on the shoulders of many pioneers and giants in this field who have afforded us the privilege of providing safer and more effective therapies to enhance physical beauty. Over the years, we have learned to reach our end goals faster, utilizing more natural approaches without necessarily having to use chemical additives or toxins.

Furthermore, as medicine has continued to advance and evolve, almost all fields have shifted from a more aggressive and invasive surgical approach using scalpels and blades to less invasive and more natural-looking esthetic procedures. The field has also shifted from using more synthetic chemicals that fill tissues toward therapies that are more natural and more regenerative. The downtime for most modern therapies can be as little as 24 hours or less. In later chapters, you'll learn exactly what happens as we age and how aging subsequently leads to facial volume loss and the dreaded droopy-face look. You'll also learn how these can be corrected naturally using amazing new technologies such as lasers and/or platelet concentrates.

As someone who has a practice devoted to esthetics, I believe in these treatments. But I also believe that you need to understand the procedures you're pursuing, so I hope you enjoy reading this book and deciding for yourself what's best for you!

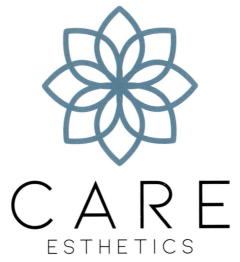

Chapter 2

Aging and the Healing Process

The aging process is no fun. Not for any of us. And that's why the doctors at CARE Esthetics love facial esthetics so much, because it allows us to turn back time, reverse that aging process, and restore a patient's self-esteem. But before we dive deep into the aging process (and how to reverse it), let's talk about regenerative medicine for a minute. Notably, many of our clinicians are gifted regenerative doctors who have treated patients with all types of complications. After all, **CARE has two main focuses: rejuvenation and esthetics.** Some of the technologies developed by our team members have been used to treat disorders like joint pain following PRF injections, osteoarthritic knees, and spinal disorders. I have witnessed patients with back pain so bad they were forced into wheelchairs walk out of the treatment room virtually pain-free mere minutes after some of these regenerative procedures. Don't believe me? Watch the video linked here!

Outcomes like this are the result of years and years of research and continuous improvement in regenerative medicine protocols. These protocols are continuously being evaluated and studied for potential further improvements. We have the privilege in the United States to work closely with some of the best universities, industrial partners, and technologies in the world to help our patients. While facial esthetics certainly does not scream "life-threatening" or "emergency," the technologies presented (such as PRF and laser therapy) have been highly researched for the treatment of complex medical disorders, many of which ARE life-threatening.

> **Note: All CARE Esthetics providers are required to purchase the most advanced technology to join and stay active members. Our society mandates that all providers are adequately equipped with the most advanced technology at all times.**

Take a look at the video linked here. ·······················>
In this case, PRF (platelet-rich fibrin) is being used to treat a foot ulcer in a patient with diabetes. For many of these diabetic patients, a lack of blood flow to the area can lead to necessary amputation if not treated. The particular focus of the CARE Esthetics clinic shown in this video is diabetic foot healing. They have literally saved hundreds of limbs with all-natural regenerative therapies in patients who were once told they needed their limb amputated. Pretty amazing stuff!

All of that is to say that this book is supported by a wide variety of research articles in medicine conducted at some of the top research facilities in the world. In fact, the protocols used for the production of PRF in our CARE Esthetics clinics are compiled in a 400-page medical textbook.[1] The very same research used to support and describe those protocols to clinicians is summarized in this book, with many before and after photographs and patient testimonials, to show our patients why these procedures are safe and effective. We take great pride in what we do, and that is why we spent the time to put this book together for you. Now let's move on to aging.

Aging Skin

Unfortunately, the aging of our skin is an inevitable process that gradually occurs as we get older. Several factors have been associated with the aging process, including both genetic and environmental factors.[2] Just like we can regenerate tissue in a foot ulcer, we can also apply the same therapeutic concepts to regenerate the skin and reduce the signs of aging.[3]

Exposure to sun, pollution, and various chemicals have been known to cause skin and/or DNA damage, speeding the aging process. A number of changes to the skin may occur as a result, including skin atrophy, telangiectasia, fine and deep wrinkles, yellowing (solar elastosis), and dyspigmentation. In addition, physical/environmental factors including poor diet, lack of exercise, caffeine intake, smoking, and drug use are also known to speed the aging process.[4] Let's discuss some of these in more detail.

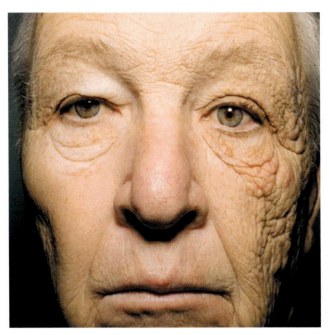

FIG 1 The facial skin of a truck driver after spending 28 years behind a window. Note that the left side of his face is severely damaged compared to the right side.

Sun

On the macroscopic level, exposure to the sun (in particular ultraviolet A [UVA] rays) is perhaps the most damaging culprit behind skin aging. Just look at Fig 1. This man, in his mid-60s, spent 28 years as a truck driver. Note the *severely* damaged skin on the left side of his face (that is, the window side) compared to the right side of his face (the shaded side). This image clearly shows how the sun affects skin, particularly skin on the face. And this is why SPF creams matter! Chapter 10 discusses the importance of cosmeceuticals (face skin care creams) for home care of facial tissues, particularly for those who spend considerable time in the sun. Next time you're deciding whether you really need that sunscreen, think of this photograph and remember why it's important!

Hydration

Another key element important for overall health but particularly for skin health is hydration. Skin dehydration is a major risk factor for skin aging. As such, many topical creams, including hyaluronic acid creams, are geared toward water retention as a modality to prevent dryness of the skin, since dryness may lead to skin cell death and flaky skin complexion. Aging skin is also related to a number of obvious demarcations of the face. Depressions in the corners of the mouth, cheeks, forehead, eyebrows, eyelids, and nose are all associated with aging and dehydration (Fig 2). Hydration is key. Similarly, too much alcohol consumption can potentially lead to additional facial aging if hydration is not taken into consideration.

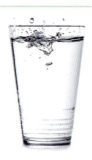

Be sure to drink a LOT of water while spending a night out: Your skin will thank you for it later!

Facial Anatomy

While this book is certainly not meant to provide in-depth knowledge of facial anatomy, patients should have a general understanding of what occurs as we age. Facial anatomy is extremely complex, but we want to highlight certain things for patients in our clinics.

The face is comprised of various tissue layers, including the skin, connective tissue, subcutaneous fat layers, as well as muscles, ligaments, and underlying bone.[3] Within this network, an array of arteries, veins, and nerves are also present. Each of these structures is prone to substantial change as aging occurs.

Younger-looking individuals have plumped muscles and tight skin with the ability to fully express themselves during facial communication, whereas aging individuals have drooping muscles and loose skin with less ability for full facial expressions. Because the face is exposed to so many external factors (for example, smoking, sun, pollution, chemicals), an overwhelming percentage of the population has at least a basic knowledge of skin care and cosmeceuticals specific to the face, much more so than any other body part. Chapter 10 handles this topic in detail and addresses

Facial Anatomy

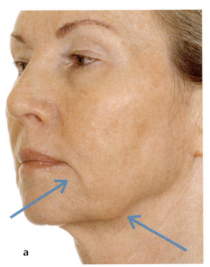
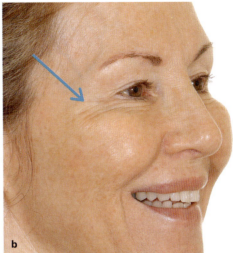
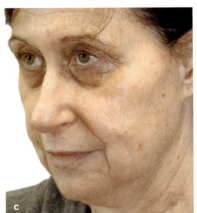

FIG 2 *(a and b)* In this 40-year-old woman, only minor changes have occurred. Crow's feet are beginning to appear more commonly, and the patient has a primary complaint in her jowl area. Now is the correct time to begin reversing these signs of aging in this patient! Waiting longer will only increase the complexity of the regenerative procedures and the number of treatments needed to reach satisfactory outcomes. *(c)* Unlike the patient in parts *a* and *b*, this patient shows advanced signs of facial aging. As a consequence, the complexity and number of treatments required to regenerate this tissue is significantly increased. At this point, discussion of reasonable expectations is required.

differences between over-the-counter facial creams and medical-grade cosmeceuticals. These alone can have a pronounced impact on your skin.

Characteristics of age-related facial changes

Regardless of how beautiful one's appearance was in youth, age-related changes such as loss of facial volume and changing features are inevitable. These are often more pronounced and specific to certain areas. A gradual loss of soft tissue occurs in the upper midface region in conjunction with a downward migration of superficial buccal fat. Consequently, as we age,

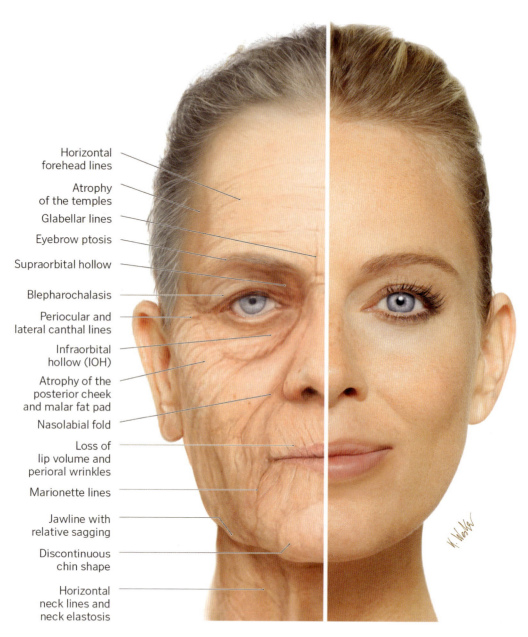

FIG 3 Typical signs of facial aging.

> **Box 1 Changes expected with normal aging[3]**
>
> - Corners of the mouth and jowls droop, resulting in a slight frown look (marionette lines)
> - Tissue around the eyes sags
> - Eyelids (upper and lower) sag
> - Tissue of the forehead drifts down, creating wrinkles and dropping the eyebrows downward with flatter appearance
> - Eyebrows sag (ptosis), giving a more angry appearance
> - Nose may elongate, and the tip may regress downward
> - Nose may develop a small to pronounced dorsal hump
> - Tip of the nose may enlarge and become bulbous
> - Youthful upside-down triangle of the face inverts
> - Skin discoloration (dark circles, superficial capillaries, pigmentary disorders) may appear
> - Skin envelope loses proportion (loss of subcutaneous fat, downward sagging of the soft tissues)
> - Glabellar lines appear between the eyebrows
> - Eyes become sunken (supraorbital hollowness)
> - Dark circles appear below the eyes (infraorbital hollowness, tear trough deformity)
> - Fat atrophies in the upper cheek region (malar fat pad)
> - Deep nasolabial folds form
> - Wrinkles appear around the mouth (smoker's lines)
> - Lip volume decreases, causing perioral wrinkles
> - Chin contour becomes irregular, dimpling and sagging

a larger proportion of soft tissue droops below the midface. While males and females tend to have different ideal characteristics when assessing overall attractiveness, and while the rate of aging varies between all individuals based on several factors (genetics, environmental factors, sex, ethnicity), there are some expected changes that occur in most people as we age (Fig 3 and Box 1).

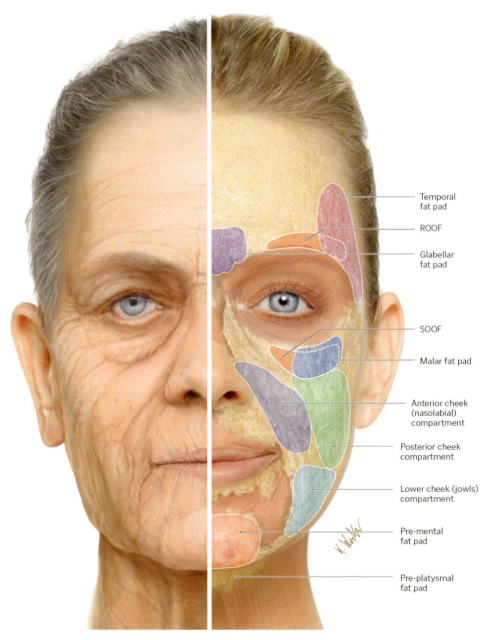

FIG 4 Fat pads found in the face and how they are affected with aging.

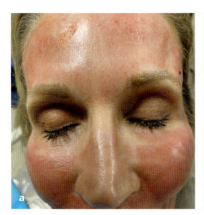 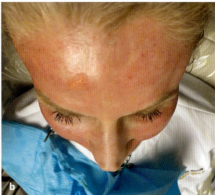

FIG 5 *(a and b)* A clear fat deficit is observed in the temple region of this patient in her mid-50s.

Subcutaneous fat and connective tissue

The most noticeable facial changes with aging typically relate to the loss of subcutaneous fat in the connective tissues of the face. This fat acts as a volumizing cushion to give skin that supple look (think plump cheekbones in younger women). Unfortunately, we lose this fat as we age, and oftentimes it simultaneously appears in other areas of the body where we do not want to have it!

Figure 4 depicts the fat pads found in the face and their loss of volume with aging. Areas that tend to wrinkle and lose volume more quickly, such as those found around the eyes (periocular region) and the mouth (perioral region) have very thin fat layers.[3] As a result, these areas often show more noticeable signs of aging, such as dark circles around the eyes or smoker/smile lines around the mouth. Patients will often complain about these two areas first, especially individuals who smoke or spend a lot of time in the sun, as their wrinkles will progress much more quickly.

Another common area where females especially lose volume over time is within the temporal fat pad of the forehead. This volume loss often gives a hollow look to this area and exaggerates the appearance of any Crow's feet. In Fig 5, for example, this lost volume in the temple region is evident in a woman in her mid-50s. Chapter 9 demonstrates what a nice difference relatively painless injections with fillers can make in cases like this.

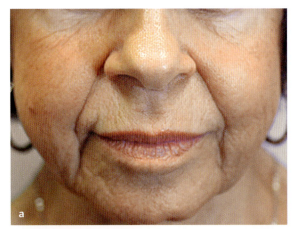

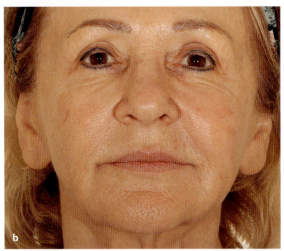

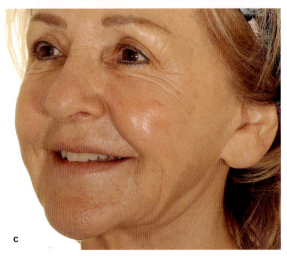

FIG 6 *(a)* Note the pronounced nasolabial folds and marionette lines requiring extensive therapy. This specific case with before and after photographs is covered in chapter 7. *(b and c)* Note that this woman has volume loss in her cheekbone area that has created deep nasolabial folds and jowls. In order to reverse her facial aging, it is best to add volume directly back into the cheekbone area, which will lift up the skin and pull it backward, thereby minimizing the depth of the nasolabial fold, instead of into the nasolabial fold itself.

The anterior cheek in the nasolabial compartment is also prone to fat resorption and volume loss over time, leaving patients with those dreaded deep nasolabial folds (so-called *marionette lines*) and droopy jowls (Fig 6). Luckily these can all be addressed with filler materials (either synthetic products such as Juvéderm/Restylane or biologic fillers fabricated from the patient's own blood; see chapter 6). However, it is important to note that these nasolabial folds often occur due to volume loss in the CHEEK, which causes the skin to sag downward, so injection into the folds themselves will not solve the problem. The correct way to address this is to put back volume where it was lost—that is, in the cheekbone area in an upward and backward motion. This will not only add youthfulness to the cheeks but also tighten the skin in the nasolabial area, smoothing those pesky nasolabial folds.

Far too often, inexperienced clinicians will want to inject where they observe these noticeable deepened lines or where the patients advise them to inject. But this is a big mistake and can often result in the dreaded "monkey" look. We see this far too often in the field! And that is why it is so important to have an in-depth and accurate understanding of facial anatomy.

Fat tissues found in the face also serve to protect it from potential external injury and to ensure a continuous supply of essential fluids and nutrients to facial tissues. In the face, areas with high fat compartments are typically well defined and homogeneous in layer. These include the cheeks, nasolabial folds, the glabella, and the jaw-chin region. In older patients, these specific tissues lose volume with age and show a resulting atrophy typically caused from reduced blood flow. This is particularly why therapies including concentrated blood (PRP and the even more potent PRF) are so effective for such conditions.

As you can see, fat isn't always a bad thing. In the face at least, fat is very important. A very thin subcutaneous fat layer exists in the area of the temples and forehead, and almost none exists in the periorbital and perioral region. These areas are therefore more prone to wrinkles and folds and tend to show the first visible signs of facial aging! Fat matters.

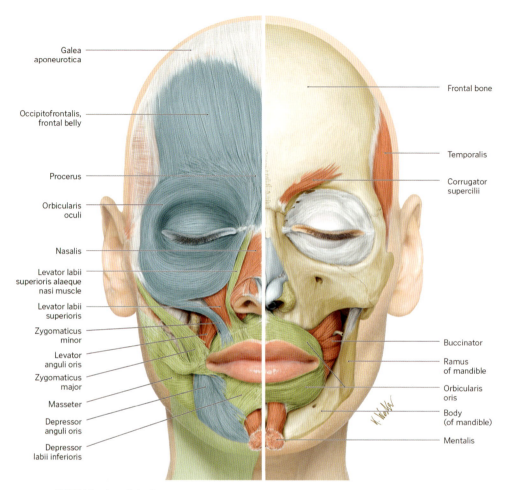

FIG 7 Muscles of the face.

Muscles of the face

Some of the strongest muscles of the body are found in the face, which houses 30 different muscles.[3] These are typically divided via three muscle planes and are thus distinguished as *(1)* superficial, *(2)* middle, and *(3)* deep (Fig 7). Muscles play an extremely important role in facial aging, especially when it comes to dynamic wrinkles caused during contraction, which can be treated with neurotoxins such as Botox. Naturally with age, these muscles become hypertrophic, permanently causing visible wrinkles that are involuntary and undesirable. The Botox section of this book in chapter 8 focuses on muscle movements and how this leads to aging.

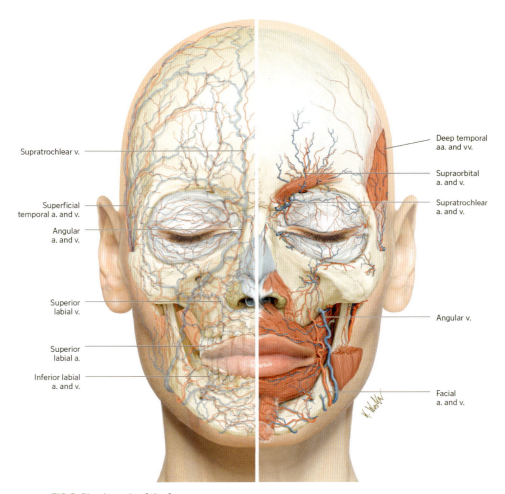

FIG 8 Blood supply of the face.

Blood supply and innervation

The importance of understanding facial anatomy is best illustrated in Fig 8. There are literally HUNDREDS of vessels (from tiny to large) that form the complex vascular network that exists throughout the face. **Therefore, any clinician injecting into the face must have a thorough knowledge of the whereabouts of all major blood vessels.** There is also a complex innervation system (nerves) that runs alongside these blood vessels (not shown).

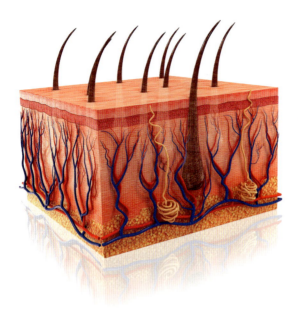

FIG 9 The epidermis is the outermost layer of the skin.

Biology of the Skin

Prior to commencing any facial esthetic regimen, it is important to have a general understanding of the various layers and cell types found in skin, since the structure and function of each layer differ. The following sections outline the various roles of skin layers and define the importance of vascularization within these tissues, providing fundamental principles and reasoning for the use of platelet concentrates.

The epidermis

The epidermis is the outermost layer of the skin (Fig 9). It is multilayered and generally considered to be subdivided into four or five separate strata. There are four important cell types in the epidermis: keratinocytes, melanocytes, Langerhans cells, and Merkel cells. The predominant cell type of the epidermis is the keratinocyte, making up 95% of the epidermal cells. Keratinocytes create keratin, which is the major structural protein of the outermost layer of the epidermis (the stratum corneum).[3] Melanocytes are the pigment-producing cells of the epidermis and are found at the basal layer, thus providing some protection of the skin from UV light. Especially when treating melasma or age spots, this layer is the one to target. When performing either a chemical peel or laser peel, the aim is to create cell turnover of this layer, thereby creating a more rejuvenated-looking layer.

The dermis

The dermis is located beneath the epidermis and is between 1.5 and 4 mm thick.[3] It is the thickest of the three skin layers and makes up approximately 90% of its thickness. The main functions of the dermis are to supply the epidermis with nutrients, to regulate temperature, and to store much of the body's water supply. The following are found within the dermis:

- **Blood vessels:** The blood vessels supply oxygen and essential nutrients to the skin and eliminate waste products. The blood vessels also serve to transport the vitamin D produced in the skin back to the rest of the body.
- **Lymph vessels:** The lymph vessels provide lymph to all tissues of the skin. These cells work to destroy any infection or invading organisms as the lymph circulates to the lymph nodes.
- **Hair follicles:** The hair follicle is a sheath that surrounds the part of the hair that is under the skin and nourishes the hair.
- **Sweat glands:** Sweat glands in the skin regulate body temperature by bringing a hypotonic solution via the pores to the surface of the skin, where it evaporates, thereby reducing the skin temperature.
- **Sebaceous glands:** Sebaceous (or oil) glands are attached to hair follicles and are found in greatest number on the face and scalp. These glands secrete sebum, or oil, that helps keep the skin smooth and supple.
- **Nerve endings:** The dermis layer also contains pain and touch receptors that transmit sensations of pain, itch, pressure, and temperature to the brain for interpretation.

The subcutaneous tissue

The subcutaneous tissue is also known as the *hypodermis*; it is the deepest skin layer, varying in thickness from a few millimeters to several centimeters. It is comprised of fat, divided by loose connective tissue into fat clusters, and separated from the underlying tissues by fascia. As previously mentioned, as aging occurs, this layer becomes thinner and thinner, giving the skin an "old" look.

Managing Facial Aging

As previously stated, the aging process is no fun. Sadly, by the time we reach our 30s, our collagen-producing cells (fibroblasts) start to lose full function, and it is estimated that we lose 1.5% of collagen production with each passing year beginning in our 20s. We often refer to our skin fibroblasts as cells that go into early retirement. Many potential factors are at play when it comes to facial aging. While initially these changes occur on the anatomical and cellular levels below the skin surface (fat tissue, muscle, and bone), eventually they become apparent on the skin.

When developing strategies to reverse facial aging, it is important for the treating clinician to understand the mechanism of tissue breakdown for a given patient (Fig 10). Was the skin damage caused by UV rays with resulting loss of collagen synthesis? Was it caused by smoking, affecting blood flow? Are wrinkles and facial folds caused by hyperactive muscles? All of this information will help the practitioner develop effective therapeutic strategies together with the patient.

Age-related changes in facial tissues most often alter blood supply, and as a result, atrophy-related deterioration will then occur. Therefore, an ability to restore blood supply, via treatment with blood concentrates such as PRF, is useful for the long-term maintenance of skin (see chapters 5 and 6). Loss of blood supply markedly and rapidly decreases fat tissue, the rate of cell division of skin cells, and collagen synthesis. Each of the above-mentioned scenarios also impairs the regenerative capacity of various tissue types and impairs the natural barrier function of the skin. Add skin dehydration to the mix, and there are even further signs of facial breakdown.

Starting with the "hot spot" regions

Many early signs of facial aging are found in "hot spot" areas of the face. These are the regions around the eyes and lips, which are more frequently clinically related to visible signs of aging. Always remember: The visible signs of the skin that are observed externally (wrinkles, skin laxity, and folds) are almost always related to an underlying cause at a deeper tissue level not clinically visible.

As mentioned previously, deep fat atrophy is a significant age-related factor for skin aging primarily caused by a decrease in blood flow (and

FIG 10 What do you think contributed to this woman's facial aging? She is currently quite tanned, so she has likely spent a lot of time in the sun. This is also evidenced by the number of age spots present and their size, especially on the right side of her face. This patient will clearly benefit more from regenerative therapy than Botox, for instance, since she still has marked demarcations and wrinkles even when her facial muscles are at rest. We'll go over the regenerative strategy we used on this patient in chapter 9 when we discuss the Bio-Lift and Bio-CARE all-natural regenerative strategies.

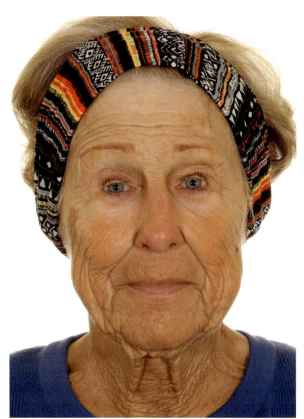

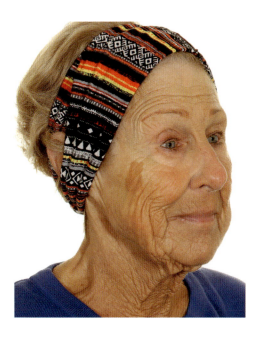

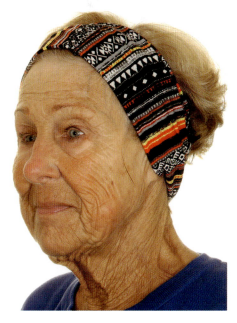

concomitant reduction in the supply of oxygen and nutrients to facial tissues). Hence, vascular degeneration is considered a major cause of the initiation of facial aging and hence why platelet therapies such as PRF have been deemed extremely effective strategies for minimizing further facial aging and potentially reversing them. These can be combined with practically all therapies and are healthy for skin before undertaking treatments in plastic surgery (ie, facelifts/necklifts) to assist with better healing. Furthermore, this is why fat grafting has become a commonly utilized strategy in facial esthetics (these are more invasive procedures performed by skilled plastic surgeons).

Common treatment options

One of the simplest treatment options to optimize overall health and particularly skin attractiveness is proper hydration. Skin dehydration is a major risk factor for skin aging, and one of the simplest modes to improve skin hydration is via the application of topical creams geared toward water retention as a modality to prevent dryness of the skin (see chapter 10).

As the body continuously ages, it undergoes many changes that directly impact the physiology of human tissues, thereby resulting in lower cellular activity and collagen production. Based on visible differences that occur with aging, a variety of treatment options have been proposed accordingly to favor a more youthful appearance. Many of the more popular options involve the injection of different forms of chemical agents/biomaterials, including Botox, fillers, and PDO threads, to name a few. These products have been made popular by extensive marketing and celebrity endorsements, which have markedly increased their popularity, and plenty of examples have demonstrated their successful use in esthetic medicine.

Importantly, however, these techniques heavily rely on normal protective mechanisms of the epidermis, which can be altered or disrupted following their use. Botox (or botulinum toxin), for example, is a toxin that generally has been effective in paralyzing muscle movement, thus limiting dynamic movements and their associated wrinkles (see chapter 8). Botox works by temporarily denervating and relaxing the muscles by preventing the release of neurotransmitter acetylcholine at the peripheral nerve endings.[5] While it is considered extremely safe and is generally advised in a protocol of repeated injections every 3 to 6 months, it does pose some secondary complications in some patients.[6,7] These complications include potential muscle paresis, including muscle weakness, brow ptosis, upper or lower eyelid ptosis, lateral arching of the eyebrow, double or blurred vision, loss or difficulty in voluntary lid closure, upper lip ptosis, uneven smile, lateral lip ptosis, lower lip flattening, orbicularis oris muscle weakness, difficulty chewing, dysphagia, altered voice pitch, and neck weakness.

Dermal fillers are also generally considered very safe, but complications are possible. In fact, dermal fillers have led to over 40 cases of blindness! While these procedures are carried out daily in facial esthetic spas and plastic surgery offices worldwide, such cases are sure to create some fear within the community. Some patients have also experienced cases of necrosis and/or allergic reactions to the products themselves. The next chapter focuses on how these and other injected or implanted materials integrate into the body.

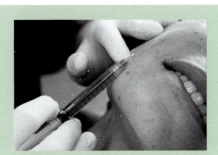

Botox and fillers have been utilized successfully in millions of patients, with very few adverse effects and a high safety profile. Proper training and use of high-quality products are of course a must.

It's no wonder why alternative, more natural options with fewer complications are constantly being investigated by researchers and clinicians who want the very best for their patients.

References

1. Miron RJ. Understanding Platelet-Rich Fibrin. Chicago: Quintessence, 2021.
2. Herbig U, Ferreira M, Condel L, Carey D, Sedivy JM. Cellular senescence in aging primates. Science 2006;311:1257.
3. Davies C, Miron RJ. Platelet-Rich Fibrin in Facial Esthetics. Chicago: Quintessence, 2020.
4. Puizina-Ivi N. Skin aging. Acta Dermatoven APA 2008;17:47.
5. Sadick NS, Manhas-Bhutani S, Krueger N. A novel approach to structural facial volume replacement. Aesthetic plastic surgery 2013;37:266–276.
6. El-Domyati M, Attia SK, El-Sawy AE, et al. The use of botulinum toxin-A injection for facial wrinkles: A histological and immunohistochemical evaluation. J Cosmet Dent 2015;14:140–144.
7. Li Y, Hsieh S-T, Chien H-F, Zhang X, McArthur JC, Griffin JW. Sensory and motor denervation influence epidermal thickness in rat foot glabrous skin. Exp Neurol 1997;147:452–462.

Chapter 3

Foreign Body Reactions

This chapter is designed to educate you to better understand the importance of health, the immune system, and what happens when foreign substances enter the body.

Many years ago, it was accepted that cells from living tissue interacted with any biomaterial implanted into the body. For example, if you needed your hip replaced with bone grafting, it was initially thought that the cells from your bone tissues (osteoblasts and osteoclasts) would interact with the newly introduced biomaterials (the titanium hip implant and the synthetically fabricated bone graft). Following this integration period, bone-forming osteoblasts would then supposedly lay down new bone matrix, and the foreign titanium hip implant would co-exist happily within your body. This is a very simplistic model that has since been amended.

Today, it is well known that the immune system (and not the cells from a particular tissue) is responsible for the integration of foreign substances.[1] Thus, when a new biomaterial is introduced into the body (say your hip implant into bone tissue), it is not bone cells that interact with the biomaterial but rather immune cells (macrophages) that gather around it. The immune system then dictates whether the biomaterial will integrate within your system or be rejected altogether. Imagine how important a healthy immune system becomes in that case!

In the scientific community, the responses to these newly introduced biomaterials were given the working name *foreign body reactions*[2] because these biomaterials are essentially foreign bodies to your immune system. Problems occur when *(1)* the biomaterial is extremely foreign to your immune cells, and the implanted material is rejected; *(2)* your immune system is not working properly and therefore rejects the biomaterial; or *(3)* your immune system is on system overload and cannot properly interact with the biomaterial.

In this chapter, let's find out what happens within your body when biomaterials are introduced.

General Health and Life Expectancy

All of us know it: Health is important. But how is the United States doing when it comes to our health? Any guesses?

Before we even begin to highlight the differences between the United States and other countries in terms of health, it is important to point out that the United States ranks among the very best in the world when it comes to developing new technology, discovering medical advancements, and educating our population. It boasts some of the best universities in the world, it produces a large proportion of the world's pharmaceuticals, and many medical procedures and breakthroughs in medicine originate here. In fact, the number of Nobel Prizes awarded to Americans matches that number awarded to all other countries combined and is nearly three times that of second-place United Kingdom (Box 1).

Box 1 Countries with the most Nobel Prize winners

- United States (375)
- United Kingdom (131)
- Germany (108)
- France (69)
- Sweden (32)
- Russia (31)
- Japan (27)
- Canada (26)

Thus, it's safe to say that here in the United States, there is no shortage of medical development, and some of the world's best doctors, researchers, universities, and hospitals are right here. This is certainly something to be proud of!

Yet still our population is one of the sickest in the world, one that takes the most medication per capita, and one with lower life expectancy compared to many similar countries (Fig 1). Over the past 30 to 40 years, life expectancy consistently rose as we improved health care and our understanding of science and medical treatments/procedures. However, in 2014, this upswing unexpectedly flattened and even declined as a result of many immune-related disorders as well as heart disease. This declining trend has continued from 2014 to 2021.

General Health and Life Expectancy

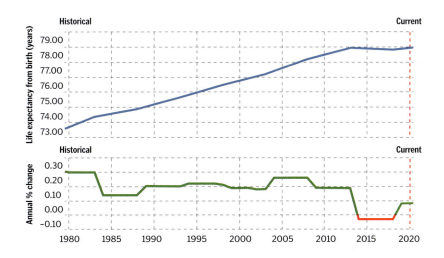

FIG 1 Life expectancy in the United States from 1980 to the present. Note that in 2014, the rise abruptly leveled off and even started to decline.

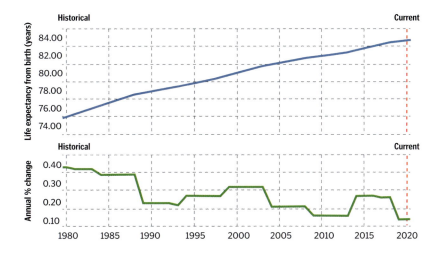

FIG 2 Life expectancy in Japan from 1980 to the present. Note the consistent increase over time with no flattening or dipping.

In contrast, Japan is known to have one of the highest life expectancies in the world. Figure 2 shows that during this exact same time period, Japan reported no such decline in life expectancy, despite the population living almost 10 years longer than Americans!

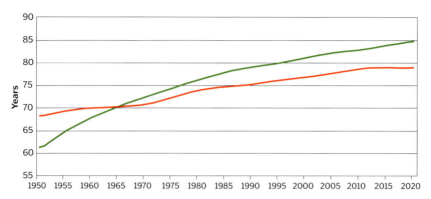

FIG 3 Comparative life expectancy between Japan *(green)* and the United States *(red)* from 1950 to 2020.

In Canada, where many of the health care guidelines and medical school education systems are adapted from the United States, life expectancy has also continued to increase over the past 5 years, greatly surpassing that of the United States.

Many Americans are unaware of these differences, and quite frankly they can be quite frightening. Just think: Only 70 years ago, life expectancy in the USA was about 7 years higher than in Japan, at 68 and 61, respectively. Over the past 70 years, this has dramatically reversed, with Japan now surpassing the USA by nearly 7 years, at 85 and 78, respectively (Fig 3). This represents a dramatic 24-year difference in life expectancy for Japan over the course of just 70 years. Think about *that* for a second. If the USA had followed the trends of Japan and Canada, we'd be living a heck of a lot longer.

Even countries that were historically known as having low life expectancy, such as China, are catching up to us, and some have even surpassed us. China has historically been known as an overpopulated country, with issues related to hunger, poor access to high-quality health care for much of the population, and higher than average air pollution due to the amount of manufacturing/exportation (especially of plastics). Despite these challenges, data over the past 60 years regarding life expectancy in China is far superior to that of the United States (Fig 4). In 1960, life expectancy was 25 years longer in the United States than in China. Today, we're neck and neck. This begs the question: How can we have the absolute best medical systems, hospitals, universities, and researchers in the world, yet be so bad at living?

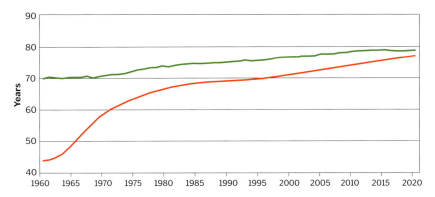

FIG 4 Comparative life expectancy between China *(red)* and the United States *(green)* from 1960 to 2020.

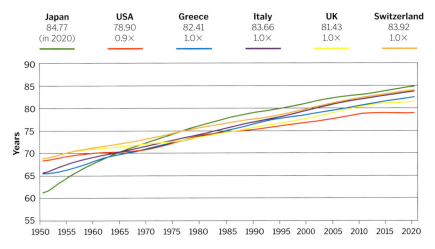

FIG 5 Comparative life expectancy among Japan, the USA, Greece, Italy, the UK, and Switzerland from 1950 to 2020.

In fact, even European countries grossly outperform us. Greece, Italy, the United Kingdom, and Switzerland each has a nearly 5-year higher life expectancy when compared with the United States (Fig 5). None of these countries show ANY decline in life expectancy, yet here in the United States we have witnessed a flattening in life expectancy over the past 5 years. What is going on?!

Think about it: At this rate, our children and grandchildren won't live as long as we do now. That's not acceptable. These trends have been alarming among the medical community, and it is clear that change is needed. So what are we doing wrong in the USA?

Evidence shows that a tremendous amount of our health woes are linked directly to the nutrition of our diets and the lifestyle we live here in the USA. These affect our immune system, so much so that our population, especially our children, bear more allergies than any other country in the world.

Allergies Among Our Children

Thirty years ago, there was relatively little known about gluten allergies. There were no tests to investigate food sensitivities. Yet today more than 30 million Americans suffer from food allergies, many of which are life-threatening.[3] There is an ever-growing population who are either gluten intolerant or gluten sensitive. Dietary restrictions among the population are becoming more and more common, and these numbers are growing more rapidly in the United States compared with any other country on the planet.[4] Again, how can this be happening in the most advanced medical community in the world?

For years experts have chimed in on this discussion, stating that improved hygiene may be linked to increases in allergies. Parasitic infections in particular are normally fought by the same mechanisms involved in tackling allergies. It has been proposed that with fewer parasites to fight, the immune system turns against things that should be harmless. Could this be true? And are we that much more hygienic than countries such as Canada, Switzerland, or the UK?

Another more common notion is that our foods are now polluted with an array of additives, more so than in any other country. Some have hypothesized that the population is not necessarily allergic to gluten but rather to the additives incorporated during its processing.[5] This may explain why certain Americans who are allergic or sensitive to gluten do not struggle as much when they eat pasta or bread in European countries. Interesting to say the least.

Another proposed culprit is the continuously increasing rise in vitamin deficiency worldwide. Vitamin D, for instance, is one of the most powerful immunomodulators, and without it, the immune system doesn't function as efficiently, thus making us more susceptible to allergies and a variety of other health-related issues that rely on a healthy immune system. While children spend more and more time indoors than ever before (mainly playing video games or being occupied with technology), the rate of vitamin D deficiency among the population has almost doubled in the past decade.[6] Vitamin D deficiency can seriously impair our immune system, especially if we are deficient for several years at a time.

Thus, while we still don't have all the answers to explain why Americans suffer allergies more than any other population in the world, it is safe to assume that our immune systems are performing at an all-time low compared with previous generations. Allergic responses and diseases related to the immune system are greatly on the rise, and this increase seems to be more linked with US culture than anywhere else on the planet.

Immune Health and Why It Matters

There has been a massive amount of research done to better understand how our immune cells interact with biomaterials newly introduced into the body.[1] But based on the previous section, we also know that the body already has issues with its immune system not functioning optimally because of the nutritional deficiencies in US culture. Even worse, that same immune system can sometimes begin to attack itself! These diseases are called *autoimmune*, and they are some of the worst in the world, including fibromyalgia, arthritis, and psoriasis, among others.

Imagine introducing a foreign substance (for example, a facial filler or hip implant) into a person who already has a shattered immune system. That biomaterial was never supposed to be there in the first place, and now the body has to deal with it. **Welcome to the world of foreign body reactions!**

Research has shown great variability in how the immune systems of various people respond to biomaterials. What might be perfectly fine in your body might not be fine in mine and vice versa. Furthermore, some implanted biomaterials are actually welcomed by the body, make immune cells happier, and improve their behavior, while others make the immune system hyperactive through massive upregulation in inflammatory markers, resulting in a ton of inflammation, not only in the local area but throughout the entire body! Imagine getting a breast implant and then noticing your hair shedding because of inflammation from a biomaterial implanted over a foot away. The body can be particular like that.

To complicate things for doctors and researchers alike, every human is unique; every human is different genetically, and every human has different allergic reactions or sensitivities to various biomaterials without advance notice to the practicing clinician. If your body has a hard time handling gluten, how is your body going to feel when it is implanted with an unnatural, synthetically derived facial filler composed of over a dozen chemicals that aims to stay active within your face over the next 12 to 18 months? These questions must be addressed before procedures are performed to minimize the chances of failure and maximize the chances of success.

If too many things go negatively, our immune systems become dysregulated, and we can encounter serious problems. This is why, for some people, when one thing goes wrong in the body, it seems like a dozen other health-related problems occur. When the immune system is dysregulated, it causes a cascade of effects. Fix the root cause, and you may just go back to normal. (Therapies to boost the immune system are covered in chapter 11.)

Macrophages

Macrophages (immune cells) are at the control center for biomaterial integration. These are your star players that you want to keep happy at all times.[1] When macrophages are in a happy state, scientists give them the working name *M2 macrophages*. When they are upset, they are given the working name *M1 macrophages*. A delicate balance exists in each and every one of our immune systems (Fig 6). If we can keep our macrophages happy, we will enjoy a lifetime of good health and happiness and likely a longer life to boot. If we keep them unhappy, we should expect an increase in inflammatory mediators and responses in our body, as well as a number of ensuing diseases down the line. And of course a lower life expectancy, as we are currently facing in the USA.

The complexity of the immune system and its relationship with health and disease underpin many of the correlations between diseases we see today. For example, diabetes is linked to a greater chance for heart attack, multiple sclerosis, and a slew of other issues. It has now been proven that periodontal disease is also linked to diabetes, cardiovascular disease, dementia, and a series of other diseases. For years medical scientists would ask: Why does that happen and what is the link? The answer is this: Bacteria occupy the pockets of space between your teeth and gums. That's normal. But when too much bacterial plaque/tartar accumulates in the oral cavity,

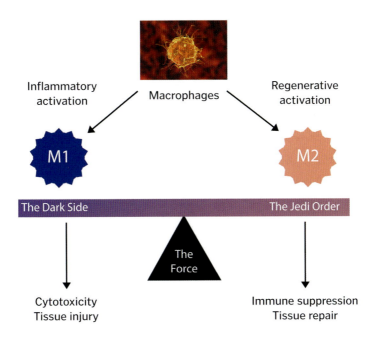

FIG 6 The delicate balance between M1 and M2 macrophages and its effect on our health and life.

the immune cells (those important cells controlling health and disease) shift from M2 (happy state) to M1 (inflammatory state), and an abundance of inflammatory cytokines and inflammation then get released into and flood the body. With this continuously circulating inflammation throughout the body, further immune cells become hyperactive and shift to an M1 state, and breakdown of other body tissue can then occur in other areas.

In fact, some time ago researchers in the dental and endocrine fields began to realize the common trend whereby people with periodontal disease also had diabetes and people with diabetes also had periodontal disease. For years researchers in both medical professions wondered: Does periodontal disease cause diabetes, or does diabetes cause periodontal disease? They figured, if we can stop one, maybe we can stop both. But after years of research, it's become clear that the answer is neither. Whether you get diabetes first or periodontal disease first, BOTH lead to greater stress on the immune system, which in turn shifts more macrophages toward that fatal M1 state (The Dark Side), which spreads inflammation throughout the body (that is, problems then occur everywhere).

Today it is well recognized that an immune system in an inflammatory state can be linked to any and all of the following diseases:

- Alopecia (hair loss)
- Alzheimer's disease
- Amyotrophic lateral sclerosis
- Asthma
- Atrial arrhythmias
- Cardiovascular disease
- Cancer
- Depression
- Diabetes
- Hypertension
- Infertility
- Multiple sclerosis
- Parkinson's disease
- Rickets
- Schizophrenia

This is why all individuals who want to live a longer and healthier life should *(1)* improve their immune cell health at all costs, *(2)* avoid biomaterials/foods that may contribute negatively to their immune system (the so-called *foreign body reaction*), and *(3)* pay particular attention to their own body and sensitivities at all times because no two individuals are the same and it becomes impossibly difficult for doctors or clinicians to predict with 100% certainty what the future may hold for any given person. In a paradigm where the country with the world's best doctors and researchers can't figure out why life expectancy is so low, we need to start paying better attention.

How Foreign Body Reactions Affect the Immune System

Let's circle back now to newly introduced and implanted biomaterials and medical devices. I like to use the common example of breast implants. For many people, breast implants are routine and lead to desired improvements in esthetic appearance. They are extremely successful in over 90% of people, have low patient morbidity, and nearly always lead to improvement in patient self-confidence. This is great news! But for some individuals, these implanted biomaterials (breast implants) can cause hair loss, immune system problems, increases in food allergies, and a number of other health-related disorders. Why does this happen in some patients but not others? We still don't know. Can we predict who may be more prone to such issues? Not really—otherwise we wouldn't be doing procedures in those prone to adverse reactions, and no one would ever have a complication.

It is estimated that 50,000 breast implants are explanted every year. This doesn't just mean the implants are removed; it means the scar tissue capsule created when the body was desperately trying to encapsulate this breast implant and keep it away from the body is also removed. Scar tissue is the body's way of creating a defensive barrier against something it perceives as being foreign and unwanted. Isn't that incredible?

Let me be clear: This is not to discourage you from getting breast implants or to encourage you to remove your current ones if you have them. This is just my way of explaining that every person is unique, and all of us need to understand our bodies if we want to have success in facial esthetics or any other medical pursuit. However, because we have seen a steady increase in food allergies and other immune-related responses in recent years, it is certainly wise to use the most natural products whenever possible. In the field of facial esthetics in particular, much improvement in facial appearance can be achieved using all-natural therapies. Future chapters will discuss how to use your body's own regenerative potential, in a 100% natural way, to regenerate your aging skin tissues and completely avoid any chance/potential for a foreign body reaction.

> **Note:** If you ever suspect you may be experiencing a foreign body reaction or any immune-related health issues as described in this chapter, seek medical attention immediately.

References

1. Miron RJ, Bosshardt DD. OsteoMacs: Key players around bone biomaterials. Biomaterials 2016;82:1–19.
2. Anderson JM, Rodriguez A, Chang DT. Foreign body reaction to biomaterials. Semin Immunol 2008;20:86–100.
3. Warren CM, Jiang J, Gupta RS. Epidemiology and burden of food allergy. Curr Allergy Asthma Rep 2020;20:1–9.
4. Gupta RS, Springston EE, Warrier MR, et al. The prevalence, severity, and distribution of childhood food allergy in the United States. Pediatrics 2011;128:e9–e17.
5. Mitchell S, Gomes A, Zelig R, Parker A. Not all grains are created equal: Gluten-free products not included in mandatory folate fortification. Curr Dev Nutr 2019;3:nzz020.
6. Mirzakhani H, Al-Garawi A, Weiss ST, Litonjua AA. Vitamin D and the development of allergic disease: How important is it? Clin Exp Allergy 2015;45:114–125.

Chapter 4

Why the Dentist?

You may be asking yourself: Why the dentist?! Why would my dentist be the best choice for facial esthetics? Well, many CARE Esthetics providers are dentists or dental physicians, and this is by design for several reasons. Before we dive deeper into that topic, let's first take a broader look at who's working in the field of facial esthetics.

There are about 6,000 plastic surgeons currently practicing in the United States. Their training includes anything from facial reconstruction to body contouring to breast/butt augmentation to liposuction. By comparison, there are roughly 250,000 dentists practicing in the United States, and their entire training has to do with teeth and the anatomy of the face, head, and neck.

In the United States, about 10% of dentists currently perform facial esthetic procedures (about 25,000 of us). This number is continuously rising and surpasses plastic surgeons more than fourfold. That's not to say that dentists are more qualified than plastic surgeons at these procedures. *Both* are qualified. But few plastic surgeons perform these minimally invasive facial esthetic procedures because they're busy with much larger reconstructive procedures—think facelifts, neck lifts, breast augmentations, nose jobs, liposuction, hair transplants, etc. In fact, many of them will focus their entire careers exclusively on one such procedure and become world-renowned experts in a single area. You can easily go to Beverly Hills and find a top plastic surgeon who ONLY does nose jobs and another who ONLY does breast implants. Some even become world experts exclusively in safe breast implant removal. Plastic surgeons are far more focused on performing larger esthetic procedures that are much more costly to the patient and thereby more profitable. They don't often enter the field of minimally invasive stuff.

Historically, many plastic surgeon offices would hire nurse practitioners or physician assistants to perform Botox injections, facial fillers with Juvéderm, and PDO threads, etc. As demand has grown, a number of these nurse practitioners have labeled themselves *injectors* to define themselves as being experts in the field of minimally invasive facial esthetics procedures conducted via injection. Just do a search on any social media platform and you'll find a slew of posts with these hashtags and even awards given out to top "injectors" in various cities! And some of these practitioners are among the world's best-trained and most successful clinicians when it comes to facial esthetics. Some of them are truly fantastic. But let's go back to the dentist for a minute.

Dentists perform dozens of injections per day, every day, starting in their early 20s, often into dark areas of the mouth, under less than perfect lighting, in fully awake and often-nervous patients. On average, dentists will perform a few hundred injections per week and a few hundred thousand throughout their careers; facial injections become routine in a matter of a few years of practice. The esthetic demands of dentistry and the artistic work that cosmetic dentists do on a daily basis (in addition to their rigorous training) is extremely relevant to the field of facial esthetics. Before I give you the lowdown on what dental training entails and why it makes the dentist perfectly suited for facial esthetics, I want to share some cool stuff on facial and physical attractiveness.

Studies on Physical Attractiveness

Professor Gordon Patzer is well known around the world for his pioneering work on physical attractiveness.[1] For years, his research focused on how the various components of the face do not contribute equally toward physical attractiveness. In fact, most of his studies focused on determining what features on a person's face led to higher or lower attractiveness scores. His research led to the notion that there is a hierarchy of importance when it comes to facial features and the attractiveness they bestow upon the bearer. As such, the five predominant features most favored on an attractive face are the following:

1. Teeth (76%)
2. Smile (75%)
3. Lips (73%)
4. Eyes (63%)
5. Nose (58%)

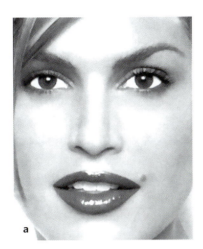
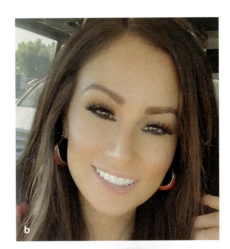
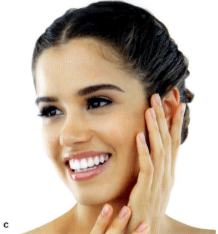

FIG 1 *(a to c)* Three women displaying attractive facial features. Note the focus on the smile and the teeth in all three images.

The top three features involve the perioral region: the teeth, the smile, and the lips. Of course dentists are well aware of the importance of esthetically pleasing results. After all, we provide the most critical work to an attractive smile, which is the most critical piece to an attractive face. Consider Fig 1. Each of these beautiful women has an attractive smile. You may then wonder: If their eyes were further apart or if their noses or ears were bigger, would they still be attractive? The answer is most likely yes. However, if they had dark teeth, crooked teeth, or missing teeth, their attractiveness would go down pretty dramatically. Just look at Fig 2. Notice anything?

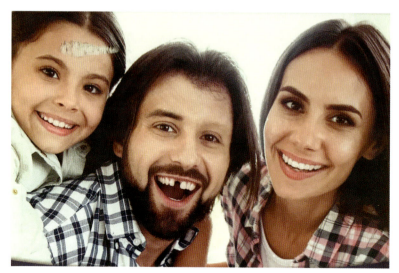

FIG 2 The perfect example to show why the teeth are so central to physical attractiveness. Did you even notice the eyebrow?

Thus, every dentist has an obligation to learn esthetics because our work, profession, and career are critically dependent on our ability to understand facial attractiveness and contribute to it. It's scientifically proven and understood now more than ever that the mouth area (including the lips) is at the center of an esthetically attractive face. This is also one of the reasons why women in general want their lips treated and filled with fillers more than any other facial area.

As dentists, we study golden ratios of tooth size and shapes and how these relate to facial proportions. We move teeth orthodontically and take x-rays to visualize where your teeth should be positioned to create an attractive smile. Many movie stars and celebrities have veneers as one of their first esthetic treatments. In older patients, we design dentures with tooth positioning and lip support in esthetically pleasing and natural-looking ways. These are things we are taught in our early 20s at dental school. Thus, further training to learn golden lip ratios and lip injection techniques and how the teeth support the lips is right up our alley.

Dental Training

I distinctly remember first-year anatomy in dental school. It was an unusual and uncomfortable experience walking into a room full of human cadavers. We often shared coursework with medical doctors in the early years of school, and in first-year anatomy our job was to learn every bone, every muscle, every nerve, every artery, and every vein in the head and neck. Each week, we would meet for a full afternoon. The medical students would be assigned weekly dissections on various portions of the body, so week after week we'd see different sections of the body being studied. We dental students would spend the same number of weeks studying in that same lab for the same full afternoon, but our sole and full focus week after week was the anatomy of the face and neck. We had to learn where every nerve of the face was located, where every artery was located, what areas were danger zones, what reactions could happen, and in what facial planes they could occur. So while year 1 for the medical doctors was focused on learning all body parts, their roles, and their anatomy, we as dentists were focused solely on mastering head and neck anatomy, becoming real experts on the face.

Dental injections

Then came the fun part in year two of dental school. After spending 1 year mastering facial anatomy, we then had to learn how to perform dental anesthetic injections. And guess who we practiced on: each other! Each of us received over 40 different injections in various areas of the mouth before we graduated to actual patients. That was certainly NOT my favorite part of dental school!

In the dental space, many of our target areas are found in the back of the mouth, often in dark areas with little light, in areas that are highly sensitive, and usually in patients who are experiencing severe tooth pain. We may have to do four to five injections per patient (sometimes even more) on 15 to 20 patients per day, every day. Even estimating on the low end, that means an average dentist performs at least 40 injections per day. Over the course of a year, that's about 8,000 injections (assuming 200 work days per year), and that's a low estimate. Over the course of a career, you're talking hundreds of thousands of injections by a single dental practitioner in dark and difficult areas that are often infected or painful for the patient. Think about the level of precision and delicacy required to accomplish that. If anyone has earned the nickname *injector*, I think dentists win by a landslide.

Consider Fig 3. Now compare that to facial esthetic injections, where the procedure is performed under direct visible light and the clinician can easily calculate their entry points and injection targets. The latter is a piece of cake for a dentist used to working in the dark.

Scale and precision

Another advantage for dentists working in facial esthetics is that we work in millimeter range and not in centimeters or inches. In dental school we are taught to use handpieces to cut teeth. (This skill is necessary to prepare teeth for restoration or veneers.) These devices typically rotate at 200,000 rpm and are attached to diamond burs to cut quickly and precisely. In our first year of dental school we were given an assortment of extracted teeth to practice on prior to using the device on any real patients. We had to cut random shapes at various depths to perfect our craft. In the beginning, cutting a shape as simple as a cross 4 mm by 4 mm was a difficult task, because teeth are not linear and we had to feel our way around their contours. But through months of daily training, each dental student becomes adept at the realities and necessities of our profession.

A dentist can very easily gauge half-millimeters. Ask any dentist to cut into a tooth at a depth of precisely 0.5 mm (not 1 mm or 0.25 mm), and he or she will easily be able to do so. Think about that level of precision. Grab a ruler and look at how short a distance 1 mm really is. To a dentist though, 1 mm is HUGE. Now imagine having to cut out a cavity on a molar in the back of the mouth through a tiny entry point in a dark area, cutting in precise increments of 0.25 mm. To a dentist, that's no problem—that's everyday, routine work.

In fact, the two professions deemed to have the absolute best manual dexterity by training are dentists and neurosurgeons. Both of these fields require hours and hours of training to develop extremely stable and accurate hands. If you want someone to be injecting something into your face, ideally you want a dentist or a neurosurgeon, and I don't think many of the latter spend much time on facial esthetics.

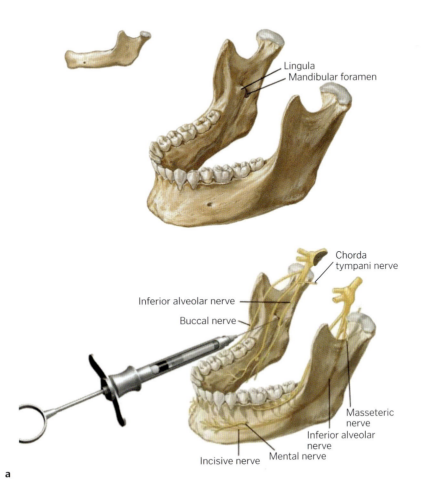

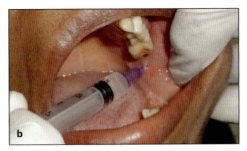

FIG 3 (a) This is a relatively common injection performed in dentistry called the *inferior alveolar nerve block*. During this injection, the goal is to target the raphe of the mandible where there is an opening (foramen). In that area, the nerve comes out of the mandible, and if it is precisely targeted, the anesthetic will numb the entire lower arch (half of the teeth in your mandible). (b) Unfortunately, this isn't the easiest area to target in the back of the mouth, the mandible being a 3D object with individualized contours. Precision is absolutely needed. To make matters worse, this area is often not visible to normal lighting, and patients are more likely to move due to increased fear of dental injections when compared with facial ones.

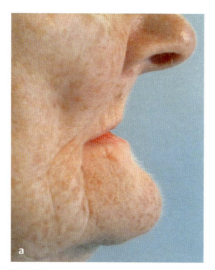 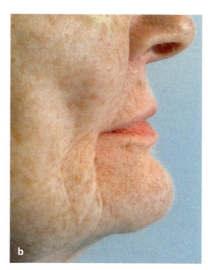

FIG 4 If you've never considered how vital teeth are to the contours of the face and mouth, just look here. *(a)* This patient was edentulous (she had lost all of her teeth), and her profile shows it. *(b)* Look how much younger and healthier she looks once her teeth are restored. Dentists spend quite a bit of time understanding lip anatomy and the means to augment and improve lip appearance as highlighted here.

Smile esthetics

Ask those who have ever had their front teeth damaged or lost how important their teeth were to their smile and facial esthetics. This is why dentists call that area the *esthetic zone*—it's literally THE most important and esthetically valuable area of the face. As dentists, tooth and smile esthetics are always on our mind, because we spend hours training in the esthetic domain to satisfy our patients.

Teeth and veneers that are just 1 mm too long or 1 mm too short look awful, and dentists know it. It's the reality we live in, especially now that patient expectations are at an all-time high. We are trained for this, and we understand the importance of facial ratios and how facial shape dictates tooth shape, including veneers. When we design dentures for someone who has no remaining teeth, for example, we have to consider proper sizing and ratios, how the lips will sit on the teeth, and how all of these features are interconnected to rebuild an attractive smile and—more importantly—overall facial attractiveness (Fig 4).

Lip esthetics

No one understands lip esthetics better than dentists do. We modify their appearance all the time simply by how we design crowns, veneers, bridges, dentures, and implants in the esthetic zone. That is why more than 25,000 dentists already offer lip fillers and Botox: because we know how to improve esthetic outcomes for our patients. We can deliver an entire "smile makeover" with veneers and lip fillers, for example, and **we understand facial harmony and esthetics better than any other medical professional**.

So when patients question why I as a dentist am performing their lip injection, I just smile, because the answer is obvious. We have some of the best hands in the medical space, we work and perform injections daily in small, dark areas, we understand facial anatomy better than anyone else, we're pros at giving precise injections, and we're responsible for the three most important esthetic areas on a person's face (the teeth, the smile, and the lips). If you want precisely 0.5cc to 1cc of Juvéderm Volbella deposited in precise anatomical landmarks in your lips, who else would you want to perform that injection?

Patients get it right away. And then we can begin to discuss the treatment plan and facial esthetic therapies together.

Reference

1. Patzer GL. The Physical Attractiveness Phenomena. Philadelphia: Springer, 1985.

Chapter 5

What Is Platelet-Rich Fibrin?

The human body is an amazing thing. Evolution has allowed it to adapt to nature, grow during specific developmental years, and heal itself when damaged, not to mention it comes preprogrammed with a variety of cells that perform different tasks via a multitude of signaling molecules whenever needed. We don't even need to think about it or tell our brain to do any of this—our bodies are on autopilot!

How We Heal

Let's say you're in the kitchen and you accidentally cut your hand while chopping cucumbers. The site automatically starts to bleed. While you're still reacting to the pain and finding a towel to stop the bleeding, your body is already beginning the repair process. As soon as the blood gets exposed to oxygen, the two main proteins found in blood—fibrinogen and thrombin—convert into a fibrin matrix. A clot then forms, the bleeding stops, and your body moves to the next stages of healing.

During these initial stages, the body uses platelets to induce the healing and clotting cascade. These cells not only assist in clotting, but they also release an array of growth factors that inform the body that it's been damaged and signal more cells to invade the area. A variety of defense-fighting immune cells then come to the rescue. These are your standard white blood cells (we call them WBCs), which are there to protect you from incoming pathogens that might try to infect the area. This is the beginning of the inflammatory process, which typically lasts anywhere from 1 to 7 days. Then comes the regenerative phase, during which incoming stem cells, fibroblasts, and in this case other skin cells assist in the repair and regenerative process. These cells lay new collagen and elastin, and a short few weeks later, *voila*, you're healed.

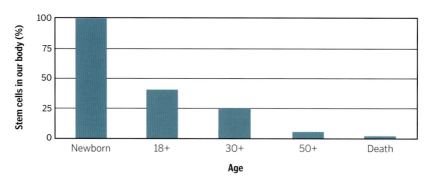

FIG 1 Number of stem cells found in the body over time. As we age, our body's ability to regenerate damaged tissue decreases as the number of stem cells significantly diminishes over time.

Over the course of this healing process for a simple cut, about a dozen cell types and likely hundreds if not thousands of signaling molecules were working in an orchestrated and perfectly timed manner. And you didn't have to do a thing. It was just part of the protective defense mechanism built into each and every one of our bodies. Incredible, right?

When we're young, healing is quick because our bodies are flush with cells that are excited and ready to go. But as we age, these cells get tired and are fewer in number. In fact, Fig 1 shows what happens to our stem cells as we age. They continuously decrease over time. By the time we hit our 30s, our bodies have a quarter of the stem cells we had as infants, and that slows our repair process considerably. Cells go into early retirement as I like to say, but still our bodies are capable of healing, just not as efficiently as when we were kids or even teenagers.

Now let's talk about the problem. What happens when the body can't heal itself? There are limits to the regenerative potential of any body, which means there are times and cases when self-renewal and healing are no longer possible. It might be from aging, it might be from a serious trauma or defect (think a serious motor vehicle accident), or it might be from a systemic issue related to healing (think diabetes). Each of these will negatively impact your regenerative potential.

Let's examine that last case, a diabetic ulcer. It is well known that individuals with diabetes don't heal as efficiently as systemically healthy individuals do. One of the major issues is the substantial decrease in blood flow that occurs as a result of the disease. This decrease in blood flow is the reason why diabetic ulcers are most commonly on the feet, because it's the furthest place away from the heart. Because blood flow is decreased, trauma to that area is not adequately infiltrated with the blood cells required for the body to naturally heal (platelets and white blood cells). The cells are still present in the body, but they can't catch the ride they need in the blood stream to get there. As a result, the healing potential is compromised, and the pesky ulcer will remain until help is sought from a medical professional. In other words, the regenerative *challenge* of the defect, created at the extremity of that person's body, was greater than the regenerative *potential* of that body to assist/facilitate healing in that area. The proper cells couldn't get there.

The same thing happens with aging (albeit at a much slower pace when compared to the diabetic individual). Eventually blood flow decreases, healing potential decreases, and the body is more prone to injury and less prone to maximum regenerative potential. Cue the platelet concentrates.

Introducing Platelet Concentrates

Over the years, scientists and clinical researchers have started to solve some of these problems by better understanding cells and the regeneration process. Cell biologists now understand the role of each cell type found in the body. We know very well that blood is composed of three main cell types: red blood cells (the cells that carry oxygen), white blood cells (the cells that fight infection), and platelets (the cells that help with clotting and regeneration). Blood also contains low levels of circulating stem cells. The problem when it comes to regeneration is that regenerative cells are found in MUCH lower concentrations when compared to other cell types. In 1 uL of blood, you could typically expect to find about 6,000,000 red blood cells, 200,000 platelets, and only 6,000 white blood cells. Our red blood cells outnumber our white blood cells by nearly 1,000 times! Figure 2 shows the breakdown of blood into its various cell types after centrifugation (high-speed spinning in a specially designed machine to separate layers).

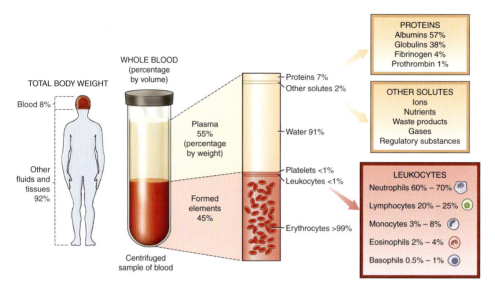

FIG 2 The various components of blood at a cellular level.

If we go back to that diabetic foot ulcer example, the issue is not just that blood flow is decreased but also that the cells needed the most to prevent infection and regenerate tissue—those white blood cells and platelets—are found in 1,000 times lower concentrations. And that's bad news for healing.

Luckily, a very smart team of researchers at the University of Miami came up with a new concept to help solve this problem. They understood that the body is an amazing organism capable of healing itself, but they had also witnessed time and time again that the body failed to regenerate itself under complex situations, many of which were related to blood flow. In the 1990s, they tested a new hypothesis. They took whole blood and thought to themselves, if we could only concentrate the cells we need—the platelets and white blood cells—in higher numbers and exclude the red blood cells we don't need, we could potentially solve some of these medical issues.

They began to draw blood from their patients using anticoagulants. Anticoagulants are safe molecules that prevent blood from clotting; this is necessary when you draw blood because, as we reviewed earlier, the body is amazing and blood will naturally clot if left to its own devices. By adding anticoagulants, the blood is prevented from clotting, and then it can be centrifuged to concentrate those important cells. A centrifugation device is a system that spins around in a circle at high speeds to separate cells based on their density. By putting anticoagulated blood into a centrifuge, it was possible to separate the less dense cells found in plasma, such as the platelets and white blood cells, from the much heavier red blood cells. And thus it became possible to concentrate cells to about 10 times their normal concentration! This new platelet concentrate could then be applied directly to the defect site to aid healing and regeneration. Genius!

This technology was given the working name *platelet-rich plasma* (PRP), and it has pioneered thousands of research papers in practically all fields of medicine. Millions of patients have been healed along the way.

Improvements to PRP

Naturally, as people learned of its healing potential, PRP became extremely popular in the early 2000s. Specifically in professional sports, all of a sudden there was a way to speed healing in multimillion-dollar athletes and get them back on the field or court faster. The orthopedic surgeons were the first to get on board, but eventually PRP found its way into other fields of medicine, eventually landing in the world of facial esthetics (see chapter 6).

However, scientists and researchers weren't done maximizing healing potential. Because remember our kitchen example. Before healing can occur, clotting has to occur. The clot is what traps those very important cells and growth factors that aid healing. And by adding anticoagulants into the PRP formulation, this clotting was actively being prevented. In the original protocols, the PRP remained a liquid formulation for injection right back into the body, and those anticoagulants were still present.

If you happen to know some people on anticoagulant therapy (for example, to prevent heart attacks), then you know that they have to be very careful to prevent bleeding. If they need surgery, oftentimes their medication will have to be adjusted beforehand. Why? Because the surgeon understands the importance of clotting during the healing phases. After all, if their blood doesn't clot, they won't heal. And in a surgical situation, that's life or death.

Let's consider a pro athlete. Say he has a meniscus tear. While the PRP injected in his knee will certainly help with healing, the anticoagulants in the formulation will actually delay clotting in that injury. As a result, the healing will not be perfectly optimized. Thus, research shifted to try to eliminate anticoagulants from PRP therapies altogether.

From PRP to PRF

Of course it wasn't as simple as removing the anticoagulants and following the same protocols, because blood naturally clots in blood collection tubes, and you'd never be able to concentrate the cells you need if the blood has already clotted. So how do you delay clotting long enough to centrifuge the blood and get the cells you need but still encourage clotting once the material is implanted in the body? Well, research in the heart transplantation and heart valve field, led to some tremendous breakthroughs here.

It is well known that if a patient has a defective heart valve that needs to be replaced, any implanted biomaterial absolutely CANNOT ever clot (or it would cause blockage of major arteries and vessels, leading to a heart attack). Therefore, researchers in that field developed biomaterials that had surface characteristics that prevent clotting to absolutely guarantee safety. Because platelets typically begin their clotting cascade on the wall surface of the collection tube, the ability to change the tube characteristics and make them more hydrophobic (water repelling) allowed a massive delay in their clotting ability. That's just what was needed!

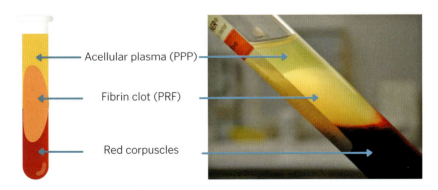

FIG 3 Illustration and clinical example of PRF showing the distinct layers.

By using this technology, blood could be collected WITHOUT anticoagulants in these newly designed specialized tubes. The blood could then be centrifuged quickly—even without anticoagulants—to separate the cell layers in the same way as PRP, and then it could be injected back into the patient as a liquid formulation WITHOUT the presence of any anticoagulants (100% chemical-free). How cool!

This new formulation was given the working name *platelet-rich fibrin*, or PRF (Fig 3). In the next chapter, we'll show you how we use it in facial esthetics!

Chapter 6

Use of PRF in Facial Esthetics

Platelet-rich fibrin (PRF) is a technology that uses your body's own powerful healing proteins and concentrated growth factors found within blood to rejuvenate skin, treat hair loss, and speed recovery.

Many patients may have heard of platelet-rich plasma or PRP, a first-generation platelet concentrate. However, as explained in chapter 5, PRP contains anticoagulants (chemical additives) that prevent clotting, which diminishes the full potential of the platelet concentrate. Recent studies have shown that PRF is up to three times more effective than previous PRP formulations. PRF encourages production of collagen, treats acne scarring, rejuvenates skin, stimulates hair growth, removes fine wrinkles, and tightens loose skin—all within the power of a simple blood draw.

In fact, if a clinic is still using PRP, one should assume that either they have not been familiarized with the newer technology of PRF or they have chosen not to keep up with advancements in the field.

> **PRP has become an outdated technology.**

Use of PRF in Medicine

Before we focus on PRF in facial esthetics, let's take a minute to appreciate what concentrated blood can do in medicine.

Remember that diabetic foot ulcer example in chapter 5 that could no longer heal due to reduced blood flow? We see such cases all the time; some of our CARE Esthetics centers are dedicated specifically to this type of healing.[1] Consider Fig 1. This 76-year-old woman has type 2 diabetes and presented to one of our clinics with chronic renal failure and severe ulcers on the back of her ankle and heel. She underwent dialysis every 2 days. The patient was also being treated for hypertension and was prescribed two types of common drugs to treat this: irbesartan (300 mg) and metformin (500 mg). She was scheduled for leg amputation after

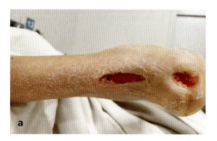 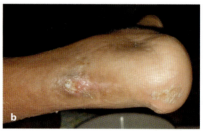

FIG 1 *(a)* Nonhealing ulcers in the foot/leg of a 76-year-old woman with type 2 diabetes and end-stage renal disease. *(b)* Healing achieved after 7 weekly treatments of PRF. PRF saved her leg from amputation.

doppler analysis (to monitor blood flow) determined that she only had 10% of normal blood flow to her leg. The patient's chronic ulcers began over 2 years prior to her presentation to our office, and they had continuously progressed. They had become infected multiple times, which is why the doctor recommended amputation in the first place. Prior to amputation, however, the patient elected to attempt therapy with PRF at one of our CARE Esthetics clinics. Following seven weekly treatments with PRF, the patient's ulcers healed, and amputation was no longer required. That's the regenerative potential of PRF!

Figure 2 shows another case treated at one of our CARE Esthetics centers in Florida. This 45-year-old woman was diagnosed with a toe melanoma (aggressive cancer requiring removal). The treatment options included amputation or skin grafting with poor prognosis due to the low blood supply to the area (remember, the toe is the furthest place away from the heart and therefore one of the more complex areas to regenerate). The patient opted to attempt the skin graft. The skin graft incorporation into the host tissue was initially diagnosed with a 50% chance of survival. Several weeks postoperative, the bandages were removed, and it was clear that the graft did not incorporate; the beginnings of bacterial infection and graft necrosis were visible. The original doctor recommended amputation. But instead the patient contacted one of our CARE Esthetics doctors, who recommended treatment with PRF. A custom-shaped graft was placed over the defect using nonstick gauze pads, and the graft was replaced weekly for 3 weeks. After 1 month, the wound healed completely. Another amputation avoided! By delivering the right cells from blood directly to the defect area, healing was possible. We just had to help the body get them there.

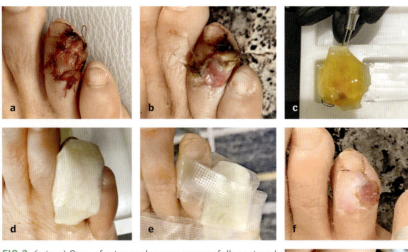
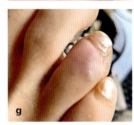

FIG 2 *(a to g)* Case of a toe melanoma successfully restored with PRF grafting after a failed skin graft attempt.

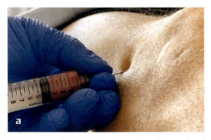
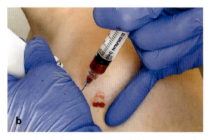

FIG 3 *(a and b)* PRF injections into this patient's osteoarthritic knees eliminated the pain entirely. PRF is a much more suitable option for knee pain compared to PRP because the clotting allows an extended release of growth factors and less bone-to-bone contact.

Another medical application of PRF is for the treatment of osteoarthritis. The patient in Fig 3 presented to our office seeking regenerative medicine therapy in hopes of avoiding surgery altogether. Following injections in both knees, the patient immediately met with relief that has since lasted months.

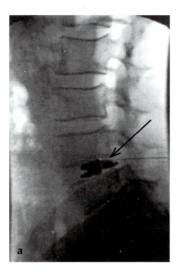
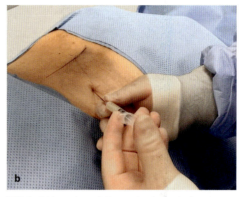

FIG 4 *(a)* Imaging of the patient's back showing an annular tear *(arrow)*. *(b)* PRF injection into the area removed the need for spinal surgery and eliminated the patient's pain.

Finally, Fig 4 shows a patient who presented to the office with a back injury that made it difficult to walk. Imaging showed an annulus fibrosus tear of the lumbar intervertebral disc. With regenerative therapy using PRF, the patient was able to walk only 15 minutes after the procedure was performed (that's the time it took for the PRF to clot!). Without this treatment, the patient would have required spinal surgery. PRF does it again!

 See the procedure and results here!

Use of PRF in Facial Esthetics

Now that we have this new and exciting regenerative agent that helps with healing, we can apply it to treat aging skin in the field of facial esthetics! **The goal for therapy with PRF is not to replace previously utilized materials but instead to offer an additional and safer modality with the ability to "regenerate" tissues naturally as opposed to fill or paralyze them unnaturally.** This certainly offers a more natural look when compared to other therapies such as facial fillers or Botox. After all, the majority of our patients want as natural a look as possible; they want to look exactly like themselves, just 10 to 20 years ago. Fortunately for them, in 2019 researchers discovered that by heat-treating PRF, it can be utilized as a regenerative filler material that lasts 4 to 6 months (similar in duration to Botox) but is still 100% natural, without a single chemical additive.

This regenerative filler is exactly what the face and skin could use as they age. Because remember, as the body ages, it undergoes many changes that directly impact the physiology of human tissues (see chapter 2), resulting in lower cellular activity.[2] A reduction in collagen synthesis as well as an associated increase in tissue degradation both lead to a net loss of facial volume, resulting in skin folds and wrinkles. By reintroducing blood-derived growth factors back to the area where tissue changes have occurred (due to volume loss, for example), not only will healing be jump-started, but facial volume will be restored, and the tissues will look more vascularized (or revived).

Therefore, several years ago it was proposed that platelet concentrates could be utilized in facial esthetics to improve collagen synthesis and restore facial tissues.[3-5] PRP was the first heavily utilized platelet concentrate shown to specifically favor wound healing when used in combination with microneedling (see below).[3-5] Because the main function of platelet concentrates is to increase recruitment and proliferation of cells and to speed revascularization/blood flow toward defective areas, PRF has only improved upon the effectiveness of PRP. Now the patient can expect *(1)* faster and better healing, *(2)* longer-lasting regenerative outcomes, and *(3)* 100% natural biomaterials. CARE Esthetics clinicians utilize the most advanced system that ensures 100% natural product safety using the Bio-PRF system developed in the United States.

Microneedling

The story behind microneedling is pretty fascinating. I'll give you the quick version.

Many years ago, a dermatologist was attempting to improve facial scarring on a dark-skinned individual who had suffered a serious facial injury. Scars often heal lighter than the adjacent skin, which means any demarcations of scars on darker skin will be particularly noticeable. Together this doctor and patient came up with the idea to tattoo the offending area with a shade similar to the patient's skin tone. By doing so, the lighter-colored scar would fade, and the hope was that her facial appearance would drastically improve. So they got out the tattoo gun, but something unexpected happened.

When the patient returned for follow-up, not only was the scar pigmentation issue fixed (the color dilemma), but the actual scar, which until then had been elevated in texture, was significantly smoothed. The only explanation was that the act of tattooing the skin with a needle actually smoothed the scar.

Intrigued by these findings, the doctor decided to do a series of similar treatments on scars like this, just without any ink (only the needling effect). And each and every time, the scars were dramatically improved and less elevated, and the skin tone was more harmonious!

Many scientific discoveries happen by accident, and microneedling is a perfect example!

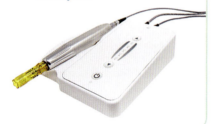

Following the success of these cases, the concept of microneedling (also known as *collagen induction therapy*) was born. It wasn't long after that a microneedling device made its way to market for scar treatment. This new device, the DermaPen, contained finer needles with an end piece typically holding 9 to 12 needles at a time to get the job done faster with better healing responses (Fig 5). Once people figured this out for scars, naturally the field expanded into treating wrinkles from aging and sun damage.

The next big discovery came when it was conceptualized that instead of putting ink into the skin during tattooing, why not add growth factors or regenerative molecules in a similar fashion? When someone gets a tattoo, a needle penetrates the skin approximately 1.5 mm, and ink is deposited into this layer, where it remains for the rest of the patient's life. But what if this same technology could be used to deliver skin-regenerative growth factors into the skin itself to further improve skin tone?

Vitamin C was one of the first materials attempted with this hypothesis, since it is known that vitamin C helps with the production of collagen, leaving patients with younger, more natural-looking skin (because younger people make more collagen). Hyaluronic acid (or HA as we call it) was next because it helps rehydrate the skin; it holds water molecules and hence leaves patients with fuller-looking faces, thereby reducing the appearance of wrinkles. From there the field naturally progressed toward using PRP/

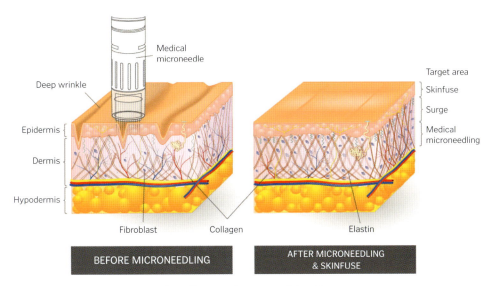

FIG 5 Microneedling pen and its effects on the tissues of the skin.

PRF, by which an array of all-natural regenerative growth factors could be utilized to more dramatically improve the skin.

Microneedling with Bio-PRF

Not all PRF is created equal—slight variations in protocol can lead to large variations in regenerative potential. In 2018 it was discovered that PRF produced via horizontal centrifugation led to much greater cell layer separation when compared with the majority of fixed-angle devices commonly used.[6] This led to the development of the Bio-PRF system, which holds many patents and trademarks for this ability to separate these cell layers most effectively and thereby concentrate as many growth factors as possible.

One of the most effective ways to get those concentrated growth factors into the skin is by microneedling. Microneedling relies on the principle of causing minimal tissue trauma to promote the formation of collagen and boost tissue repair. The DermaPRF pen, released to market in 2022, is an electrically powered medical device that delivers a vibrating stamp-like motion to the skin, effectively creating a series of microchannels. The

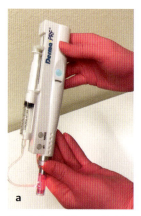 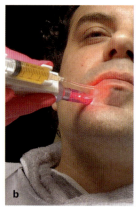 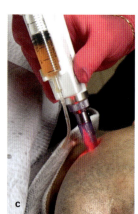

FIG 6 *(a to c)* DermaPRF device in use.

microneedles are spring-loaded and can be adjusted in height to achieve penetration depths ranging from 0.25 to 2.5 mm depending on the task. For instance, if the skin on your forehead is thinner than on your cheek, the depths can be adjusted accordingly. Greater depths may also be used to treat uneven skin like scars or stretch marks. As these microchannels are created, they are simultaneously filled with PRF. Much like a tattoo gun, the device pushes the product (in this case, PRF) into the skin to facilitate facial rejuvenation via growth factor release[7] (Fig 6).

Box 1 Indications for microneedling

- Skin resurfacing
- Reducing/removing fine lines and wrinkles
- Improving uneven texture, tone, and color of the skin
- Managing photoaging or sun damage
- Reducing skin laxity
- Improving scars
- Treating acne scarring

Microneedling with PRF is an extremely safe skin-resurfacing therapy and results in minimal damage to the skin. The patient downtime is usually only 24 to 48 hours, which is considerably shorter than other comparable methods of facial rejuvenation. In addition, microneedling has a lower risk of side effects, making it an ideal treatment choice, particularly for patients with thin, sensitive, or darker skin.[8] It is also especially effective in smokers and other indi-

FIG 7 *(a and b)* Following microneedling with Bio-PRF, a general glow may be observed after a single session.

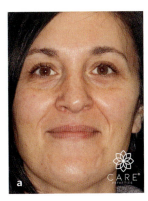
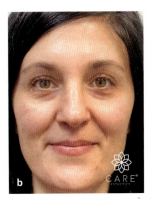

viduals who have been exposed to external pollutants, as they often require the regenerative potential of PRF to assist in their healing and recovery.[9]

Microneedling boasts several advantages[10]:

- Short healing times when compared with other modalities (typically 24–48 hours)
- Can be utilized on all skin types
- Well tolerated by patients
- Minimal risk of postinflammatory hyperpigmentation or bruising because the needle depth penetrates the skin a maximum of 2.5 mm
- Encourages the production of collagen
- No chemicals or additives

Figure 7 shows some before and after photographs with this technology, and an accompanying short video highlights the use of microneedling with PRF for face and neck tightening. This field is continuously improving and will only continue to do so. Below are some frequently asked questions and their answers.

What can I expect after a microneedling procedure?

Typically the skin will appear red (similar to a mild sunburn) for 24 to 48 hours. Almost immediately after the procedure, your skin will feel tighter,

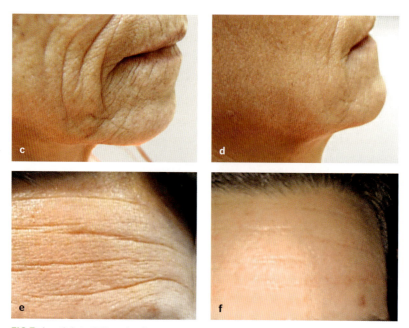

FIG 7 *(cont) (c to f)* Note the dramatic improvements in skin texture as well as fine lines and wrinkles when several treatments are performed.

with greater improvements usually observed within 3 days. Depending on your skin color and condition, you may completely heal within 24 hours post-therapy, especially if an appropriate posttreatment skin care regimen is followed.

How long do the effects of microneedling last?

Within 24 hours, patients will begin to notice an immediate glow of the skin. Collagen production will reach its peak about 2 to 4 weeks post-therapy, and these effects should last for up to 6 months.

How long does the procedure take to perform?

The procedure generally takes about 30 minutes total. It takes 15 minutes or so to draw and centrifuge the blood in the Bio-PRF system. Once the layers are fully separated and the PRF layer can be drawn up, it is then microneedled into the treatment area. It takes approximately 10 to 15 minutes to complete the entire face and neck. All of our treatments also

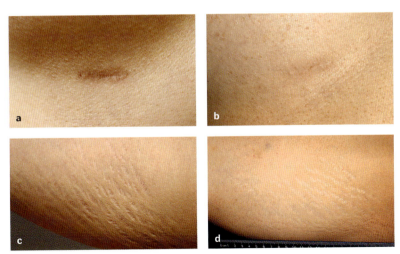

FIG 8 *(a and b)* Before and after photographs of a scar below the breast area following treatment with microneedling and PRF. Note the substantial improvement in skin texture. *(c and d)* Before and after photographs demonstrating improvement in substantial and pronounced stretch marks following microneedling with PRF as well as subcutaneous liquid-PRF injection.

focus on tightening skin laxity of the neck, which we offer complimentarily with all of our facial treatments.

How does the procedure work?

Typically, a small sample of blood is collected the same way as in a blood lab, and the tubes are immediately placed in a Bio-PRF centrifugation system to concentrate cells and growth factors up to 10 times higher than what's typically found in whole blood. This super-concentration of blood is then topically applied to the face, and the microneedling device pushes it into various deeper layers of the skin to promote tissue regeneration.

> **Microneedling with PRF is a go-to treatment modality for smoothing fine lines, wrinkles, and acne scars, and it favors a healthy, glowing skin texture.**

Can microneedling be used on other body parts?

Absolutely! In fact, many of our therapies use microneedling with PRF for the treatment of body scars or stretch marks. Have a look at Fig 8, and book a consultation to discuss your personal situation.

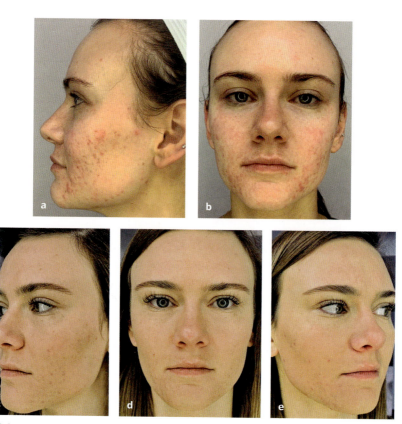

FIG 9 *(a and b)* This teenage young woman was basically unwilling to leave her home due to the psychologic impact of her acne. *(c to e)* Three treatments of microneedling with PRF was all it took to resolve her issue and change her life.

Microneedling with Bio-PRF for Acne Treatment

The use of microneedling with PRF for acne treatment has become a large portion of our overall clinical activity. Acne can be quite debilitating both physically and emotionally, especially for young teenagers. Most commonly, young individuals are prescribed pharmacologic therapy such as Accutane or other drugs that cause some secondary toxicity (to the liver especially). Years ago, it was hypothesized that because acne is a skin infection caused by bacteria, by using the PRF fraction highly concentrated in white blood cells (the cells that fight infection), a higher probability of healing could be achieved. This has now been well studied and confirmed in the literature.[11]

Figures 9 and 10 illustrate how powerful the body's immune system can be if encouraged correctly with concentrated PRF. After all, it is always

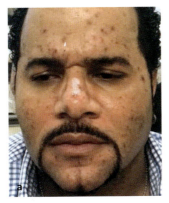
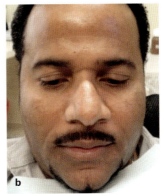

FIG 10 *(a)* Acne persisted throughout the life of this man in his 30s to the point where he assumed he'd have to live with it for the rest of his life. *(b)* He was offered microneedling treatment with PRF, which totally cleared his skin.

best to avoid medication or drug therapy when all-natural regenerative modalities are available instead.

Delivering More Liquid-PRF via Small Papule Injection

One of the benefits of Bio-PRF is that in more troublesome areas, it can also be injected via extremely small needles because of its liquid consistency. This is particularly beneficial when patients have specific areas that are more wrinkled and/or damaged. The three areas most requested by patients are:

- Fine lines and wrinkles around the eyes (squinting lines)
- Glabellar lines between the eyebrows (we call these our "number 11s")
- Nasolabial fold lines (the lines that extend from the corner of the nose to the corner of the mouth)

In such cases, it is advantageous to deliver more growth factors to local areas (a larger amount). With small papule injection, it becomes possible to deliver up to five times more volume into these areas prior to microneedling. Consider Fig 11 and the accompanying video to appreciate just how tiny these needles are.

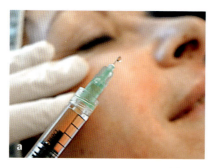
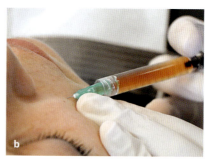
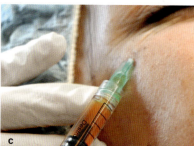

FIG 11 *(a to c)* Injection of PRF prior to microneedling. Look how tiny the needle is!

So how does this even work? Basically, liquid-PRF is injected directly under the skin to create a sort of swimming pool of growth factors below the surface prior to microneedling. Then, the stamping motion of the microneedling device fills all the channels with PRF. By utilizing this combination approach of both modalities, one can significantly improve fine lines and wrinkles in these trouble areas (or any area that the patient would like to specifically address). Following are a couple frequently asked questions and their answers.

Is the use of needles more painful than microneedling alone?

No! The procedure is virtually painless because a topical cream is applied to numb the area beforehand. The needles used are all microneedles and hardly even visible to the eye.

How many treatments are required to rejuvenate the skin?

Like with other treatment modalities that aim to regenerate the skin instead of fill it, generally speaking two to three treatments are better than one.

When using a chemical dermal filler, for instance, the area is immediately filled with that chemical, which then slowly dissipates over time. When using PRF, the body goes through a regeneration process where it begins to repair itself and produces its own collagen. Therefore, maximum results are typically seen 2 to 3 months post-therapy, as the body continues to make collagen for you, as opposed to simply filling it with a synthetic derivative.

Using PRF can lead to better, more natural, and longer-lasting results that are certainly healthier for you, but the result is not as immediate as with traditional fillers. However, the addition of 10 times the number of regenerative cells found in normal blood means more growth factors, more ways for the tissue to regenerate itself, and more ways to reduce postoperative time using what is naturally found in your own body. That's a win-win.

Utilizing Liquid-PRF for Hair Regrowth

It is currently estimated that over 80 million Americans suffer from hereditary hair loss with an esthetic desire to reverse the condition. This has been reported in both men and women. While a number of treatment options have been proposed, one currently used therapy that is minimally invasive and has been shown to be effective at treating early-onset hair loss is the use of platelet concentrates. Originally PRP was proposed as a means to halt progressive hair loss and, in many cases, to improve hair density, but the advancements in PRF have only improved the game.

Two techniques may be used to administer PRF into the scalp to treat alopecia: injection or microneedling. With either technique, the scalp is numbed prior to treatment.

Box 2 Aims of PRF treatment for alopecia

- Restore local microcirculation
- Provide growth factors and fibrin to the affected area
- Slow the programmed process of follicular involution
- Stimulate the hair's environment with needling effect
- Complement other treatments (hair care, medication, etc)
- Use as an adjunct to other hair treatments such as PDO threads

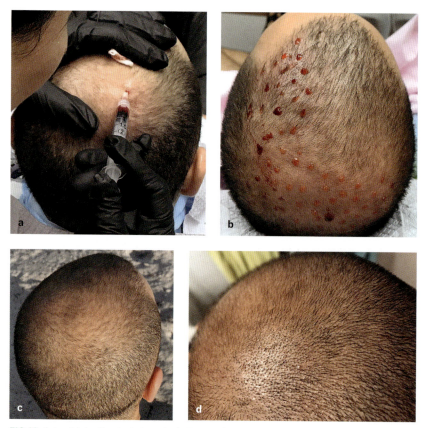

FIG 12 *(a to d)* Injection technique for hair growth with PRF. Note that the technique involves performing several PRF injections under the scalp about 1 cm apart. Over the course of several months, hair regrowth is noticeable.

Tips for successful treatment

Patients should make sure the hair is properly shampooed and detangled prior to their session. The hair must be free of any hair wax, gel, or spray.

Protocol

Patients typically follow a series of three appointments to deliver PRF 1 month apart for 3 months. Hair typically begins to grow by 1 month, with maximum hair growth observed at the 3-month mark. Figures 12 to 14 illustrate some sample cases.

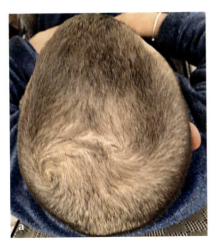
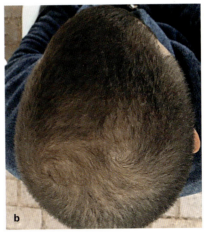

FIG 13 *(a and b)* Note that it is best to begin treatment when hair shedding or balding is mildly observed. Experts estimate that by the time you realize you have begun balding, nearly 50% of your remaining hair is left. Hence the need to perform therapy as soon as you notice any changes from normal.

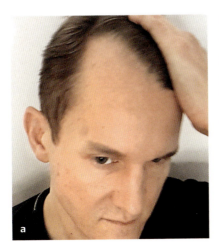
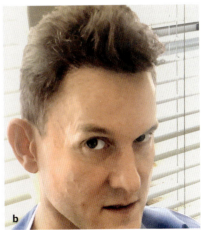

FIG 14 *(a and b)* PRF is often combined with hair transplants to improve their success rate. Note the nice outcome when these treatments are performed by skilled CARE Esthetics providers.

Creating an Entirely Biologic Filler

One of our cornerstone treatments at CARE Esthetics is the use of an all-natural facial biologic filler (the Bio-Filler). This trademark belongs to CARE Esthetics because the scientists who comprise our CARE team developed the Bio-Filler within their research labs to bring this technology to fruition.

What makes this Bio-Filler so special is that it overcomes one of the only limitations observed with both PRP and PRF: their relatively short half-life (or the time it takes to break down and be absorbed back into the body).

PRF aims to restore and regenerate tissues, but it has a hard time acting as a true "filler" because its use is associated with a relatively fast resorption time (typically 10–14 days). This means that within 2 weeks of treatment, those growth factors are released, regeneration starts, and collagen is produced over the next 6 months. But that nice "filled" look is not as apparent as with synthetics.

Certainly PRF is effective in improving skin tone and texture, but deep folds generally require a more permanent and volume-stable material. Because of this, traditionally many clinicians would combine PRF with synthetic fillers such as Juvéderm or Sculptra to achieve the look the patient was expecting. However, as we've learned so far in this book, any synthetic filler has the potential to cause a foreign body reaction because chemicals are then at play. Therefore, for individuals who have a history of complications with synthetic materials, who are prone to allergies, or who simply desire a more natural alternative, something better was needed, so the researchers got thinking again.

In 2019, a novel breakthrough was made, and methods were discovered to extend the working properties of PRF.[12] When researchers biologically heated plasma albumin, the resorption properties of PRF were found to be drastically extended from a standard 2-week period to more than 4 to 6 months. This concept was introduced to the market as an all-natural biologic facial filler (Bio-Filler) that could last as long as some synthetic fillers but without any of the chemicals.

Clinical use of the Bio-Filler

The Bio-Filler has been utilized in thousands of cases across our hundreds of offices here in the United States. But it has also become quite popular internationally, specifically in Europe and South America, because the entire world prefers to use a more natural alternative. Figures 15 and 16 show what's possible with the Bio-Filler, available on a daily basis in our clinics, and following are a few frequently asked questions and their answers.

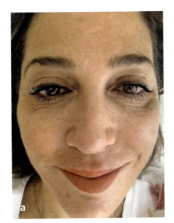
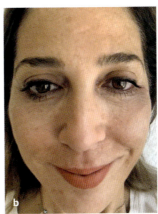

FIG 15 *(a)* This woman has lost considerable volume under her eyes in the tear trough area. *(b)* Note the better skin texture under the eyes after a single injection with the Bio-Filler.

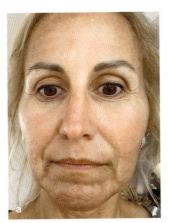
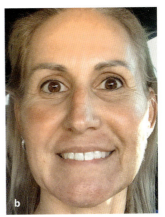

FIG 16 *(a and b)* Photographs of a woman in her mid-40s before and after receiving Bio-Filler injections. Note the loss of volume around both her temples and cheekbones. In her case, treatments combined Bio-Filler injection with microneedling and laser therapy (this Bio-CARE protocol is described in more detail in chapter 9). Note the dramatic change that occurred when these areas were filled. This was the first time in the history of the field that such results could be obtained by offering all-natural therapies using PRF, Bio-Filler, and laser therapy in combination.

This book could be filled with case after case of before and after photographs showcasing the possibilities with various PRF treatments. If you are interested in seeing more patient results, simply visit us at CARE Esthetics or join our social media pages. We'd be more than happy to go over different procedures with you.

How is the Bio-Filler made?

Following 2 years of extensive research, the Bio-Filler technology was launched as a 100% all-natural filler. To process Bio-Filler, PRF is heat-treated to drastically extend its working properties. The entire preparation takes about 25 minutes, and the results generate a long-lasting natural regenerative look.

Does the Bio-Filler still regenerate tissues?

Yes, absolutely! In fact, the same technology is also used for much more serious and complex disorders such as diabetic ulcers, knee injections, and spinal injections. Research on the Bio-PRF technology has actually been more widespread in medicine, and it's just recently that it's been introduced to clinicians in facial esthetics. The Bio-Filler protocol has resulted in positive outcomes and been proven to induce collagen synthesis when implanted within the superficial and deeper layers of skin. This technology has the special ability to form a stable clot following heating, which provides superior volume enhancement when compared to standard PRF.

What are other advantages of the Bio-Filler?

Beyond its extended half-life, the Bio-Filler's main advantages include the following:

- 100% natural and chemical-free
- Safe for individuals with allergies and autoimmune diseases
- Offers a more natural look
- Generally healthier for all patients

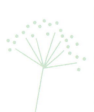

> If you are a first-time facial esthetics patient, you may want to consider going 100% natural with CARE Esthetics.

Certain types of artificial facial fillers may lead to problems for individuals with allergy complications and various forms of autoimmune limitations. Our natural and scientifically precise methods are safer for our patients with these health concerns. And they can be combined with laser therapy for all-natural regeneration, as discussed in the next chapter.

References

1. Miron RJ. Understanding Platelet-Rich Fibrin. Chicago: Quintessence, 2021.
2. Dimri GP, Lee X, Basile G, et al. A biomarker that identifies senescent human cells in culture and in aging skin in vivo. Proc Natl Acad Sci 1995;92:9363–9367.
3. Kim DH, Je YJ, Kim CD, et al. Can platelet-rich plasma be used for skin rejuvenation? Evaluation of effects of platelet-rich plasma on human dermal fibroblast. Ann Dermatol 2011;23:424–431.
4. Redaelli A. Face and neck revitalization with platelet-rich plasma (PRP): Clinical outcome in a series of 23 consecutively treated patients. J Drugs Dermatol 2010;9:466–472.
5. Na JI, Choi JW, Choi HR, et al. Rapid healing and reduced erythema after ablative fractional carbon dioxide laser resurfacing combined with the application of autologous platelet-rich plasma. Dermatol Surg 2011;37:463–468.
6. Miron RJ, Chai J, Zheng S, Feng M, Sculean A, Zhang Y. A novel method for evaluating and quantifying cell types in platelet rich fibrin and an introduction to horizontal centrifugation. J Biomed Mater Res A 2019;107:2257–2271.
7. Clementoni MT, B-Roscher M, Munavalli GS. Photodynamic photorejuvenation of the face with a combination of microneedling, red light, and broadband pulsed light. Lasers Surg Med 2010;42:150–159.
8. Fernandes DJO, Clinics MS. Minimally invasive percutaneous collagen induction. Oral Maxillofac Surg Clin North Am 2005;17:51–63.
9. Amer M, Farag F, Amer A, ElKot R, Mahmoud R. Dermapen in the treatment of wrinkles in cigarette smokers and skin aging effectively. J Cosmet Dermatol 2018;17:1200–1204.
10. Litchman G, Nair PA, Badri T, Kelly SE. Microneedling. Treasure Island, FL: StatPearls, 2020.
11. Davies C, Miron RJ. Platelet-Rich Fibrin in Facial Esthetics. Chicago: Quintessence, 2020.
12. Gheno E, Mourão CFAB, Mello-Machado RC, et al. In vivo evaluation of the biocompatibility and biodegradation of a new denatured plasma membrane combined with liquid PRF (Alb-PRF). Platelets 2021;32:542–554.

Chapter 7

Lasers in Facial Esthetics

Lasers are another technology that has gained tremendous momentum in recent years. Why? Because they're incredible!

Think about this: Just 30 years ago, cataract surgery in your eyes was a gruesome experience with lengthy downtimes. The ophthalmologic surgeon had to use blades to cut through various portions of your eye, correct the issue, and suture your eye back up.

Not only can this procedure be performed better with a laser, but lasers are much more precise and do not require any surgical blades or cutting. Most impressive is that clinical research has figured out exactly which laser wavelengths target respective areas of the eye using various intensities. A laser procedure is therefore faster to perform, safer, and it leads to better outcomes and less downtime. What a brilliant technology!

Laser devices, however, are extremely expensive, ranging from $200,000 to upward of $1 million. While a medical practice such as an ophthalmology clinic wouldn't survive without one, the average procedure may cost $10,000, easily justifying the cost of the device. But in a facial esthetic spa where the average procedure costs a tenth of that, the high price tag of the laser device can become a problem. Luckily, due to increased demand and production in recent years, laser costs have been decreasing, making them more affordable for smaller clinics performing less complex procedures. The average facial esthetic laser may run anywhere from $150,000 to $250,000. This remains a VERY expensive piece of equipment, but the use of lasers in facial esthetics is essential. Many med spas will remain stuck in the past, offering Botox and fillers in small treatment rooms, if they do not invest in better, necessary equipment like this.

Twenty years ago, laser treatments were limited to ablative therapies (that is, they removed certain layers of the epidermis or dermis) and were much more invasive, with long downtimes and often less-than-optimal results. The latest technologic advances in this space, however, have expanded the capabilities of laser wavelengths to indicate nonablative therapies as well, which has flown open the door for facial esthetics. Today, lasers are on

Chapter 7 ■ *Lasers in Facial Esthetics*

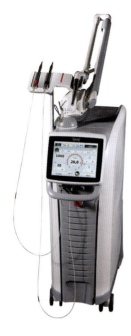

FIG 1 At CARE Esthetics, we believe in the absolute best technology, and that means a Fotona laser in each clinic. You, like all of our patients, will receive treatments identical to what you see celebrities getting on social media.

the market for various indications including scar revisions, pigmented lesions, vascular lesions, hair removal, facial resurfacing, facial rejuvenation, fat ablation, and laser lipolysis. In fact, even some of the most influential celebrities, such as Kim Kardashian, have posted videos on social media documenting their laser therapy protocols. In her case, she was treated with the same Fotona laser system that is found in every CARE Esthetics clinic across the country (Fig 1).

What Are Lasers Anyway?

Laser is an acronym for **l**ight **a**mplification by **s**timulated **e**mission of **r**adiation, which articulates precisely how light is produced. Lasers emit an electromagnetic radiation with its own characteristics that differ from common light: It has a single wavelength that is collimated (has parallel rays) and directional with high concentration of energy.[1] The main goal of treatment is to put energy into the skin tissue at a precise wavelength to stimulate collagen formation, therefore making the skin tighter and younger looking. These lasers can also selectively target specific chromophores to treat age spots, veins, hair, moles, dark circles around the eyes, etc.

One concern with lasers is safety. When we talk about safety with respect to lasers, we mostly worry about their potential for causing eye injury. Safe lasers include laser pointers used to point to a screen during a presentation and to keep your cat entertained chasing the light on the ground. These are lower-energy lasers at work. But when we want to create enough energy for, say, nonablative facial esthetic therapies, higher-energy lasers are required. The great thing is that more energy can be delivered more precisely, and in medicine we want the most precise device possible, hence the high price tag of these devices.

The video linked here demonstrates the power and potential of lasers, illustrated through the removal of a pigmented lesion on the skin (age spot). This procedure was done in less than a minute and was virtually painless. A specific wavelength of laser was utilized to precisely target the chromophores causing the discoloration. Stuff like this is routine for our clinicians.

It's important to understand that lasers can interact with tissues in many different ways. The extent of the interaction between the laser and the tissue is dependent on many factors related to the laser itself (wavelength, applied energy, peak power, power and energy density, exposure time) as well as the optical characteristics (reflection coefficient, absorption, and scattering) and thermal properties (thermal conductivity and thermal/heat capacity) of the tissue.[1] The absorption of laser energy can be attracted to water molecules, proteins, or pigments. The absorbed portion of the laser radiation can produce photochemical and/or photothermal effects depending on the wavelength of the laser radiation and nature of the tissue.[1] All of that is to say that a medical laser is not a simple device to use, and extensive and mandatory training and knowledge are required to operate one effectively and with the margin of safety patients deserve. If you are pursuing laser treatment, you want the best-trained and most talented providers with proper education, like those found at CARE Esthetics.

Laser Therapy in Facial Esthetics

Carbon dioxide lasers (CO_2 lasers) were the first ablative laser used for skin resurfacing, originally developed by Richard Fitzpatrick.[2] Despite early promising results, a long healing period (about 2 weeks) was needed because full reepithelialization was necessary following therapy. Nevertheless, the technique achieved satisfactory results and encouraged industrial development of new laser alternatives with a more focused and precise energy application to create less intense side effects.[3] Today we are much better able to control laser intensity and thereby avoid such complications and lengthy downtimes.

The two most well-studied laser wavelengths are what a lot of patients call "YAG" lasers (short for yttrium aluminum garnet). There are many different types of YAG lasers, but erbium YAG (Er:YAG) and neodymium YAG (Nd:YAG) are the two most researched in medicine and most commonly used in facial esthetics.

The following therapies use the photothermal capabilities of the Er:YAG and Nd:YAG lasers to convert and initiate the formation of new collagen in tissues to support tissue tightening of the face, neck, and lips. The Er:YAG wavelength (2940 nm) is best for cutting tissues because it is attracted to water, whereas the Nd:YAG wavelength (1064 nm) is best utilized for vascular and pigmented lesions because it is less attracted to water. There is obviously much more science behind how these therapies work, including their ability to target specific chromophores and tissues, but that could take and has taken up entire textbooks.[4] Below we simply discuss various treatment options available to patients with lasers.

Laser peels

While chemical peels have been utilized for decades as a resurfacing agent aimed at removing the upper epithelium, the use of laser peels offers a much more controlled and precise therapy. Chemical peels essentially vaporize a layer of skin, thus leaving the skin with a nice refreshed look once it heals. They are also known to improve hyperpigmentation and reduce fine lines and wrinkles. Laser peels can do the same with less downtime, and they eliminate any hypersensitivities caused by the chemical irritants. The laser peel aims to remove either part of or the entire epidermis, leading to exfoliation of the skin, removal of superficial lesions, and regeneration of a new epidermis. In a nutshell, **treatment with lasers is much more specific and controlled with less irritation compared to chemical peels.**

Today there is a growing trend toward resurfacing treatments using the Er:YAG laser.[5] Figure 2 demonstrates the results of one such laser peel with the Fotona laser system, which is the only Er:YAG/Nd:YAG dual-wavelength laser system available on the market to date. Chapter 9 showcases many cases like this using all-natural combination treatments, including our

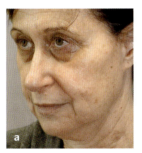 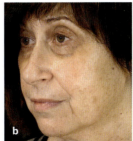 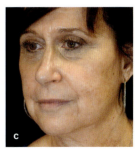

FIG 2 *(a to c)* Photographs taken before and after five treatments with SmoothLase intraoral applications (described later in this chapter) and a light fractal peel using an Er:YAG laser. Note the dramatic change in skin tightening and reduction in skin laxity as well as improved skin brightness in c, taken 30 days after the laser peel.

signature Bio-Lift and Bio-CARE treatments available at CARE Esthetics clinics.

Pigmented lesion/mole removal

To effectively treat pigmented lesions, a good diagnostic and histopathologic classification of the lesion is necessary. With this information, the lesion can be categorized according to the depth of the target pigment distribution: epidermal, dermal, or a combination of both.[6] The success of the Q-switched (QS) lasers in the realm of pigmented lesions is based on the ability of these lasers to selectively target melanosomes situated within melanocytes (melanin-forming cells) and keratinocytes. The goal of therapy is to target melanosome-specific damage using the absorption of high-energy, nanosecond laser pulses specific to that target.[7,8] Long-pulsed lasers in the millisecond domain can also be used to target epidermal and dermal pigments (dark spots) found in larger clumps, such as those in nested melanocytes or confluent melanin in the epidermis.[9] Alternatively, for superficial lesions, the Er:YAG laser can be used to ablate superficial age spots as presented in Figs 3 and 4. Age spots like this are especially common in individuals who live in southern states (Florida, Arizona, or southern California), who live at high altitude (Utah, Colorado), or who simply spend a lot of time in the sun.

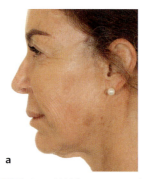 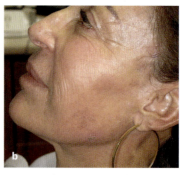

FIG 3 *(a and b)* These images demonstrate the time-lapse effects of age spot removal. Laser treatment may form small skin scabs over the treatment area, which fall off about 1 week after the procedure. Afterward, the originally darkened areas are considerably lightened or gone entirely.

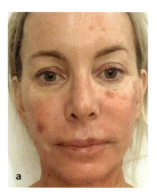 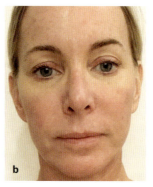

FIG 4 *(a and b)* Before and after photographs demonstrating successful laser removal of very noticeable age spots on the patient's cheeks.

Hair and vein removal

It's been over 20 years since it was discovered that lasers could be used effectively for hair removal by selective photothermolysis of hair follicles using a normal-mode ruby laser. As with other laser therapies, novel laser sources were thereafter introduced.[10] The target is the melanin pigment present in the hair bulbs. The purpose is to destroy the bulb, which leads to permanent epilation (hair removal). Only the bulbs that are in the anagen phase (the active phase of hair growth) are destroyed. In the following catagen and telogen phases, the hair gradually detaches itself from the bulb, which is why several treatments are required to fully remove hair

FIG 5 *(a and b)* Use of the Nd:YAG laser to remove spider veins.

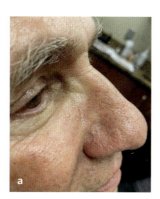
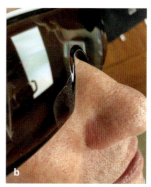

(as the hair is in different stages of growth). Similarly, the Nd:YAG laser in particular is very effective to target veins (Fig 5). The linked videos here demonstrate the use of the Fotona laser for both hair and vein removal. These procedures are always wow factors for patients because they take only a few seconds and the hair and/or veins can be removed instantaneously!

Intraoral rejuvenation of deep nasolabial folds and marionette lines

The last decade in particular has seen some of the most amazing advancements in laser therapy. One such advancement was the technology developed by Fotona called SMOOTH mode, which utilizes the Er:YAG wavelength with lower nonablative energy delivered in pulses. SMOOTH mode is based on the controlled emission of a sequence of low-power pulses inside a very long pulse that results in temperature increase inside the skin without any surface ablation. Instead of causing ablative injury, each pulse is thermal and able to travel deeper and deeper into tissues with each stacked pulse. Time plus temperature equates to thermal injury to the tissue, and the body responds by producing tighter and thicker collagen bundles. And voila! The skin is tightened as a result. No outward injury and no scabs, which means a quick recovery period. Not surprisingly, this SMOOTH mode technology has since been used for a number of procedures from surface skin texturing to tightening dark circles under the eyes, improvements in lip texture and plumping of the lips, and even tightening the vaginal canal to improve sexual function in females.

This same laser therapy can also be used to treat those deep nasolabial folds and marionette lines that everyone complains about as they get older. But there's one caveat: Instead of directing the laser energy onto the skin itself, the laser energy is directed toward the nasolabial fold from INSIDE the mouth. The clinical researcher who discovered this reported several advantages:

1. The procedure could be performed entirely inside the mouth with no external redness. The tissue is still tightened and collagen formation still takes place, but no visible sign of any treatment can be detected.
2. The skin inside the mouth always heals faster than the skin of the face. After all, skin tissue recovers best in moist environments. That's why we always recommend some type of skin lubricant like Aquaphor following any external treatment. The skin on the inside of the mouth (mucosal tissue) is naturally moist and therefore heals faster as a result, which means shorter recovery periods following this intraoral protocol.
3. Perhaps most importantly, **the skin on the inside of the mouth is thinner than that of the face.** Therefore, the laser energy can actually penetrate more effectively and deeply into the nasolabial folds and marionette lines, offering better results.
4. The procedures can be done in combination. Thus, if a patient is really dissatisfied with their nasolabial folds, they can receive targeted treatments both intraorally and extraorally, offering double the laser energy to the same area.

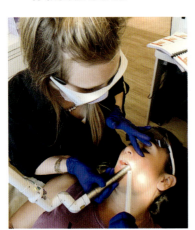

This intraoral protocol was given the working name SmoothLase (Fig 6), and the linked video here demonstrates how it works. Figures 7 and 8 illustrate the results of this protocol.

FIG 6 One of our CARE Esthetics clinicians performing intraoral rejuvenation of nasolabial folds with SmoothLase technology.

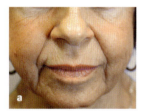 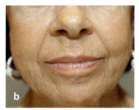 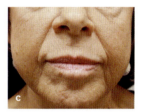

FIG 7 Case example demonstrating the use of the intraoral SmoothLase protocol to treat deep nasolabial folds *(a)*. *(b)* Results at 30 days after treatment. *(c)* Results at 42 months after treatment, with no touch-up therapies performed in between. Note that the patient should have received updated treatments but still demonstrates visible improvements nearly 4 years after treatment.

FIG 8 *(a and b)* Photographs taken before and 30 days after laser treatment performed in conjunction with PRF application. These results were achieved after just one treatment.

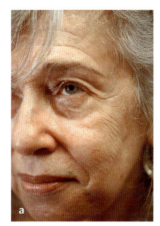 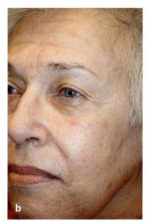

SmoothEye protocols

Fotona also adapted this technology to improve the typical bags found under the eyes. The SmoothEye procedure takes only 15 minutes to perform, and the results are dramatic (Fig 9).

LipLase

This technology can also be used to augment the lips. While this may not give the sort of volume desired by many young women (think Kim Kardashian or Angelina Jolie), the laser energy is able to improve collagen formation when a series of treatments are performed, resulting in slightly fuller and more supple lips (Fig 10). This is definitely a more natural look than some of the other lip treatments out there.

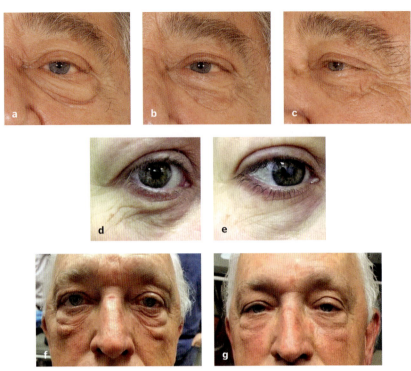

FIG 9 *(a to c)* This patient was bothered by his visible eye bags, so we performed a series of three treatments every 21 days. Note the improvements that occurred over time. *(d and e)* Before and after photographs of a woman in her 50s. *(f and g)* Note the immediate tissue response after therapy in this 75-year-old man.

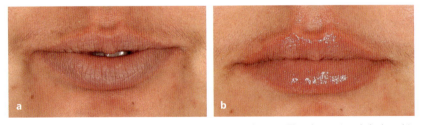

FIG 10 *(a and b)* Photographs before and after LipLase therapy. The change is subtle, but this all-natural boost in collagen does add volume to the lips to create those fuller lips young and middle-aged women seek.

Combination approaches

Chapter 9 discusses the use of lasers in combination approaches with PRF using our Bio-CARE protocols, which are the majority of treatments we do here at CARE Esthetics.

Treatments Based on Patient Condition

One of the benefits of having a high-end professional laser system in the office is the ability to treat a multitude of conditions. Here we will review some of the most common procedures done either using laser therapy alone or in combination with other therapies. For all of these conditions, laser therapy plays a pronounced role in treatment.

Fine lines and wrinkles

While fine lines and wrinkles are not a medical "condition," their elimination is the most common procedure desired by patients. Many options are available depending on the cause of the wrinkles themselves (hyperactive muscle, sun damage, smoke damage, dehydration, etc) as well as their severity. Several facial esthetic strategies can be implemented from anti-aging agents to regenerative therapies aimed at minimizing the onset of fine lines and wrinkles. These can also be performed in conjunction with more conventional therapies such as muscle paralysis (Botox) or basic fillers (Juvéderm, Sculptra, etc).

When patients desire the regeneration of their tissue with an end goal of having radiating and glowing-looking skin, PRF in combination with laser therapy is ideal. Of course this can also be combined with Botox, PDO threads, and fillers as well. Chapter 8 examines some of these combination therapies.

Acne and acne scars

Treatment for acne and acne scarring is the second most commonly performed procedure within our offices. Studies have shown that approximately 80% of the population suffers from acne at some point in their

> **Important application:** This same technology is also used to successfully treat sleep apnea. In patients with sleep apnea, the soft tissue of the palate has expanded and often blocks airway space, resulting in difficulty breathing when the muscles are at rest (during sleep).[11] This laser technology has been used to tighten the soft palate, thereby creating more airway space. This alone can often resolve snoring, and almost immediately posttreatment, patients often report that they can breathe better.

lives, often resulting in scar formation, pits, or changes in skin texture. Acne can visually be detected in several forms and varied severity, affecting all skin types at all ages. Furthermore, acne and its scars may cause just as much emotional damage as physical discomfort in some patients, especially teenagers with dimples resulting from past inflamed blemishes. As explained in chapter 6, many teenagers are steered toward receiving various drugs such as Accutane to resolve acne. These are quite harsh pharmaceuticals/chemicals, and the ability to treat acne using all-natural approaches is certainly beneficial from a health perspective.

At CARE Esthetics, treatment for acne and acne scars always uses a combination of laser therapy and PRF to first target the bacteria and then fight it off with those accumulated white blood cells. See chapter 6 for case examples showcasing the dramatic results possible *without* drugs.

Rosacea and visually observable facial veins

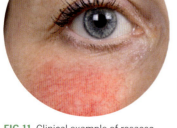

FIG 11 Clinical example of rosacea.

Rosacea is usually a chronic condition characterized by redness of the face, most commonly observed around the cheeks, nose, and forehead (Fig 11). Patients also develop visible blood vessels (apparent veins) on their face (termed *telangiectasia*). Lasers are the treatment of choice for this condition, often in combination with microneedling with PRF (Fig 12).

Even in its mildest of forms, rosacea often leads to patients expressing dissatisfaction with the red, blue, or purple visible veins on the face (especially when present on the lower face). Laser therapy is a go-to therapy to remove small vessels without discomfort.

Sun damage and melasma formation

Sun damage (age spots) can be one of the most prominent factors progressing facial aging. Brown "patches" appearing on the face are caused by too much melanin production (termed *melasma*) following excessive sun exposure, resulting in unnatural facial discoloration. Sun damage also exposes facial tissues to the harsh damage of UV light, resulting in a rapid loss of skin elasticity and decreased ability to produce collagen. Anyone living in

FIG 12 *(a and b)* This patient presented to the clinic with a chief complaint of literally painful skin. Her official condition was rosacea with acne bumps that appeared to be seasonal and infected. She was treated using a combination of laser therapy and microneedling with PRF. *(c and d)* After three treatments, her issue was almost entirely resolved with no remaining pain experienced in the area. Watch her video testimonial here!

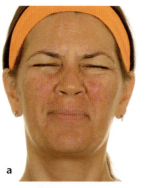
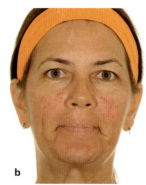

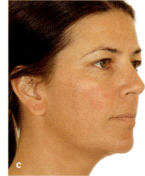
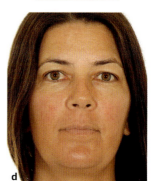

a sunny state or at high altitude (closer to the sun), or simply anyone who enjoys spending a lot of time outside, should consider a daily skin care regimen with high-SPF sunscreen (more on this in chapter 10).

Treatment with laser therapy, PRF, and microneedling can bring substantial improvements in skin texture and facial aging caused by sun damage. Melasma formation is best treated with lasers and/or certain pigment-correction serums. In such cases, a consultation is required to determine which facial treatment approach will be best to treat your skin depending on the severity of your condition and your skin type.

Mole removal

Moles also spring up as we age. These are easily removed via laser therapy that is virtually painless. Your doctor will remove the mole in a controlled layer-by-layer fashion until the mole is entirely gone. Much like dark spots, these are easy skin treatment procedures to eliminate the condition and greatly improve patient satisfaction and facial esthetics.

Chapter 7 ■ *Lasers in Facial Esthetics*

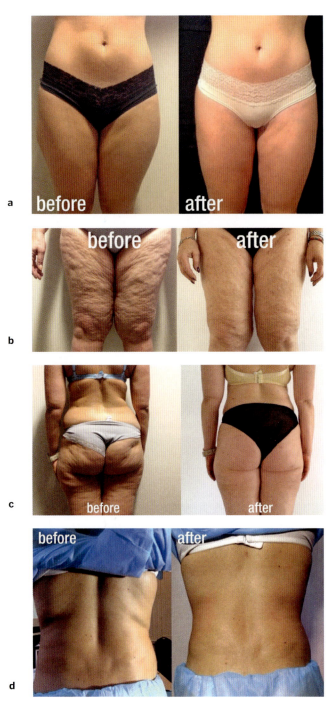

FIG 13 Case examples showing the results of full-body TightSculpting in the abdomen and thighs *(a)*, legs and butt *(b and c)*, and back *(d)* using laser therapy.

Full-body TightSculpting

Laser therapy is also used very successfully for full-body skin tightening, fat ablation, and general improvements in skin appearance with Fotona TightSculpting. The technology is much the same, whereby a combination of Nd:YAG and Er:YAG lasers are utilized in specific protocols to help tighten the skin. Figure 13 shows some dramatic before and after photographs to demonstrate the results possible with this novel approach.

> **Book your free consultation!**
>
> Lasers offer an extremely wide variety of treatment options. When you aren't sure, always seek more information and feel free to book a complimentary consultation with any of our staff members at CARE Esthetics. We have access to hundreds of research articles, resources, textbooks, and of course clinical experience that can help you learn more. Every patient is unique, and we want you to choose for yourself what is right for YOU.

References

1. Mahamood RM. Laser Metal Deposition Process of Metals, Alloys, and Composite Materials. Philadelphia: Springer, 2018:11–35.
2. Goldman MP, Fitzpatrick RE. Cutaneous Laser Surgery: The Art and Science of Selective Photothermolysis. St Louis: Mosby, 1994.
3. Chen K-H, Tam K-W, Chen I-F, et al. A systematic review of comparative studies of CO_2 and erbium: YAG lasers in resurfacing facial rhytides (wrinkles). J Cosmet Laser Ther 2017;19:199–204.
4. Davies C, Miron RJ. Platelet-Rich Fibrin in Facial Esthetics. Chicago: Quintessence, 2020.
5. Avci P, Gupta A, Sadasivam M, et al. Low-level laser (light) therapy (LLLT) in skin: Stimulating, healing, restoring. Semin Cutan Med Surg 2013;32:41–52.
6. Kilmer SL, Garden JM. Laser treatment of pigmented lesions and tattoos. Semin Cutan Med Surg 2000;19:232–244.
7. Goldberg DJ. Benign pigmented lesions of the skin: Treatment with the Q-switched ruby laser. J Dermatol Surg Oncol 1993;19:376–379.
8. Raulin C, Schönermark MP, Greve B, Werner S. Q-switched ruby laser treatment of tattoos and benign pigmented skin lesions: A critical review. Ann Plast Surg 1998;41:555–565.
9. Brazzini B, Hautmann G, Ghersetich I, Hercogova J, Lotti T. Laser Tissue Interaction in Epidermal Pigmented Lesions. Oxford: Blackwell Science, 2001.
10. Grossman MC, Dierickx C, Farinelli W, Flotte T, Anderson RR. Damage to hair follicles by normal-mode ruby laser pulses. J Am Acad Dermatol 1996;35:889–894.
11. Shiffman HS, Khorsandi J, Cauwels NM. Minimally-invasive combined Nd:YAG and Er:YAG laser-assisted uvulopalatoplasty for treatment of obstructive sleep apnea [epub ahead of print 25 February 2021]. Photobiomodul Photomed Laser Surg doi: 10.1089/photob.2020.4947.

Chapter 8

Botox and Dermal Fillers

Botox and dermal fillers have been used successfully in facial esthetics for decades. While many of the specific products are chemically or synthetically derived and may cause foreign body reactions, their use in facial esthetics oftentimes leads to excellent long-term results. This chapter describes the synthetic compositions and mechanisms of action of various fillers and Botox and details their individual benefits and potential complications, with before and after photographs highlighting their use.

Botox

Botox is certainly the most popular minimally invasive facial product on the market. Originally approved by the FDA in 2002, Botox has an annual revenue of around $4 billion! In fact, its initial manufacturer, Allergan, was just acquired by the pharmaceutical company AbbVie in June 2019 for $63 billion (note that this acquisition includes the entire Juvéderm brand as well as CoolSculpting). This price tag gives you an idea of the global value of Botox and Juvéderm.

What exactly is Botox?

Botox is a neurotoxin (botulinum toxin) produced by the bacterium *Clostridium botulinum*, a gram-positive anaerobe.[1] It functions by blocking presynaptic nerve synapses, preventing the release of the neurotransmitter acetylcholine at the neuromuscular junction. In more basic terms, it stops neurons from sending signals to each other. This results in a decrease in muscle activity and weakness.[1] This means that Botox can effectively paralyze facial muscles, thereby reducing the appearance of wrinkles during facial movement. When utilized long-term, Botox can dramatically decrease facial aging.[2] The most common treatment areas include the glabellar lines, forehead lines, frown lines, and crow's feet.

Botox has been popularized by celebrity figures and is now the most widely used cosmetic treatment in the world, with millions of patients receiving routine treatment globally.

Typically, the muscle relaxant feature will last anywhere from 3 to 6 months, but this varies considerably among patients. The more often and the longer time period a patient has been receiving Botox treatment, the less of an effect it will have (because the body develops neutralizing antibodies against it). For first-time users, it could take 3 to 7 days to fully see the effects of Botox.

History of Botox

Botulinum toxin was first discovered in 1897 as the product of the anaerobic bacterium *C botulinum* and as the causative agent of botulism food poisoning. The development of a purification method for the toxin began in 1944 and led to crystallization of the type A serotype.

Investigations on the potential clinical applications for botulinum toxin were initiated by A. Scott in 1968. It was first approved by the FDA in 1989 for involuntary muscle disorders but then was granted full approval in 2002 for esthetic applications. The following types of Botox A are now commercially available:

- Ona botulinum toxin A (BOTOX, Allergan)
- Abo botulinum toxin A (Dysport, Ipsen)
- Inco botulinum toxin A (Xeomin, Merz)
- Pra botulinum toxin A (Jeuveau, Evolus)
- CS-BOT (Chiba Serum Institute)
- Chinese BTX-A (Prosigne, Lanzhou Biological Products)

Clinical uses of Botox

The upper face has traditionally been the most popular location for Botox treatment. The appearance of the upper face revolves around the positioning and shape of the eyebrows, and this must be considered at all times when treating the surrounding area.

Vertical frown lines: The brow

The muscles comprising the brow or glabellar complex include the corrugator supercilii, the procerus, and the medial part of the orbicularis oculi.

FIG 1 *(a)* Placement of Botox injections for treatment of vertical frown lines. *(b and c)* Clinical examples of results following Botox injection.

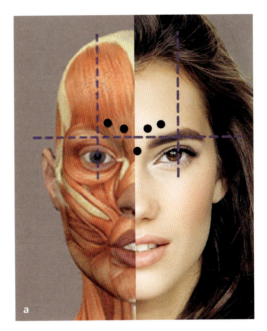

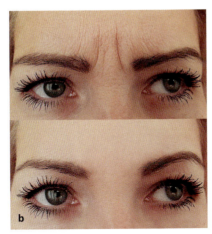

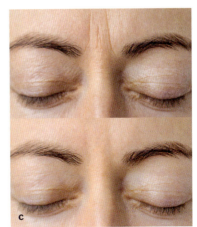

Action of these muscles is responsible for the creation of vertical frown lines known as the "11s." Treatment of this area must always take into account the interactions among these closely related muscle fibers.

Typically, multiple injection sites (five to seven) are required. All points should be 0.5 to 1 cm from the upper orbital rims and internal to the midpupillary lines (Fig 1).

Note that gender differences must be taken into account when treating this area because the male brow has a straighter appearance compared to the arched brow of females.

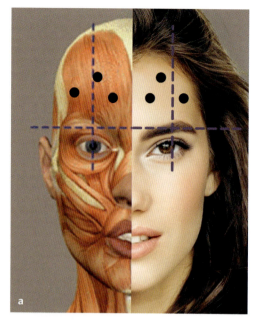

FIG 2 *(a)* Placement of Botox injections for treatment of horizontal expression lines. *(b and c)* Clinical examples of results following Botox injection.

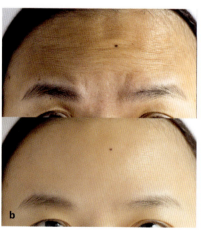
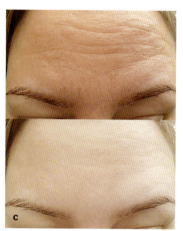

Horizontal expression lines: The forehead

Horizontal forehead lines arise as a result of the underlying frontalis muscle, which acts to elevate the eyebrows. Patients may exhibit a single deep furrow or may be afflicted by multiple smaller rhytides (fine lines and creases).

A total of six to eight injection sites are recommended in the forehead below the hairline. The points should form a slightly curved V-shape in women (Fig 2) and should be straight in men if applicable (depending on their brow position).

FIG 3 (a) Placement of Botox injections for treatment of crow's feet. (b) Clinical example of results following Botox injection.

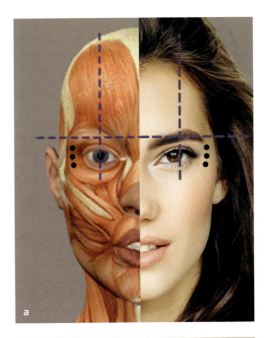

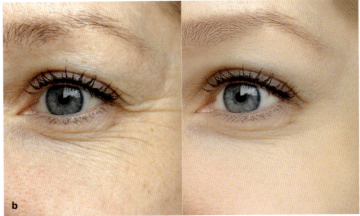

Lateral orbital wrinkles: Crow's feet

Crow's feet arise as a result of underlying muscle hyperactivity in the orbicularis oculi muscle as well as photoaging. We often ask patients to squint their eyes like they're in a sandstorm to discover the depth of these lines. The wrinkles may also appear when smiling.

If you have dry eyes, prominent eye bags, or morning eyelid edema, you should notify your practitioner.

Typically three to five injection sites are needed per side (Fig 3). Lower doses are generally required in this region.

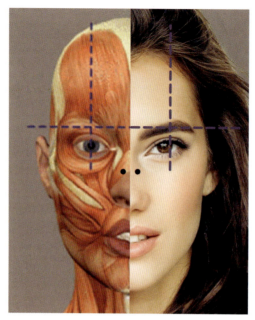

FIG 4 Placement of Botox injections for treatment of bunny lines.

Paranasal downward radiating lines: Bunny lines

These lines are visible on either side of the nose and result from wrinkling or scrunching of the nose due to the action of the transverse portion of the nasalis muscle. Low-dose, superficially administered injections are usually successful to improve the appearance of these lines (Fig 4).

They tend to be treated in conjunction with the glabellar complex rather than in isolation, specifically the transverse nasal lines, across the nasal bridge, which result from procerus contraction.

Lower face

The lower face is not as straightforward of a treatment area as the upper face, and generally patients should expect greater variability in results, with typical combination treatments being performed. Aging in the lower face has much more to do with volume loss than wrinkles, and thus facial fillers, PRF, and lasers are likely better candidates for treatment in this area. That being said, a combination of Botox with any of the aforementioned treatment options has been well established but should be administered

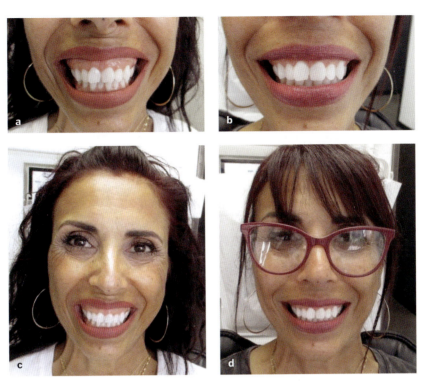

FIG 5 *(a to d)* Use of Botox to relax the muscles that make a gummy smile overly visible. Botox relaxes the muscles above the upper lip, leaving an esthetically pleasing result.

on a case-by-case basis. Botox can be used for correction of downturned corners of the mouth, dimpled chin, necklace lines, and platysmal bands. Figure 5 shows how it was used to treat a gummy smile.

Summary of Botox treatment

Although Botox is one of the most potent toxins known today, it is a very safe drug if used appropriately by well-trained professionals. Despite its overall safety, the use of Botox is not altogether free of complications. The most common complication tends to be short-lived muscle inactivity of untargeted muscles. Few people are directly allergic to Botox.

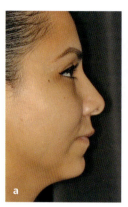 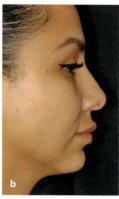 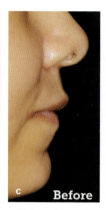 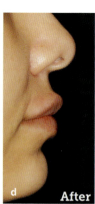

FIG 6 *(a to d)* Photographs before and after the injection of 1.5cc of Restylane Kysse in the lips and 2.0cc of Restylane Defyne in the chin.

Dermal Fillers

Dermal fillers are the second group of commonly used synthetic derivatives in the "minimally invasive facial esthetic" portfolio. The main fillers that are approved by the FDA fall into four classes:

1. Hyaluronic acid (HA): Juvéderm, Restylane, Perlane, Belotero, Stylage, Teoxane, etc
2. Poly-L-lactic acid (PLLA): Sculptra
3. Calcium hydroxylapatite (CaHA): Radiesse
4. Polydioxanone (PDO) threads

HA

HA is a linear polysaccharide that is a common component of normal skin, where it forms part of the extracellular matrix of the dermis. Because it is negatively charged, it attracts large amounts of water and therefore maintains hydration. In its native state, it is degraded by the body in 1 to 2 days. However, if it is stabilized chemically, the resulting product takes several months to be degraded by the body (typically 4 to 8 months, but it can be even longer if engineered to do so).[3,4] Variation in the particle size of HA also changes its viscosity, and this will influence the indications and the areas to be treated. For example, finer lines or scars are more commonly treated by smaller particle sizes, whereas larger particle sizes are used for deeper lines and folds.

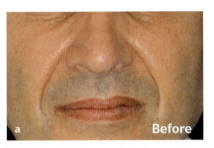
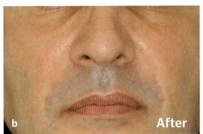

FIG 7 *(a and b)* Photographs before and after the injection of two syringes of Restylane Defyne into the nasolabial folds using a 25G cannula and one syringe of Restylane Lyft in the medial cheek area.

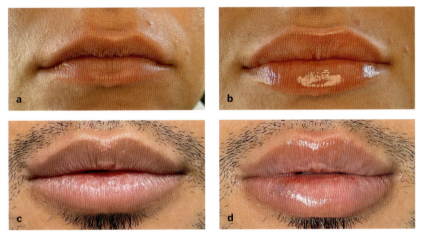

FIG 8 One commonly performed procedure is lip augmentation. *(a and b)* Photographs before and immediately after the procedure. Note the minimal redness following treatment. These treatments are often combined with dental veneers to drastically improve facial attractiveness. As reviewed in chapter 4, the teeth, lips, and smile are the three most prominent features on the scale of facial attractiveness. *(c and d)* Another clinical example of lip augmentation using Juvéderm Volbella.

Main indications of HA
- Volumizing the cheeks, lips, chin, and scars
- Reshaping the lips, chin, and jawline
- Rejuvenating the hands, neck, nasolabial folds, and marionette lines

HA can also be injected into the tear trough area, glabellar lines and crow's feet, nose, brow, and temples to increase volume at those sites. Figures 6 to 8 demonstrate the common uses of HA fillers with excellent long-term results.

PLLA

PLLA (known as Sculptra in the industry) is a semipermanent soft tissue filler with effects that can last up to 2 years.[5] It is considered a deep tissue regenerator, and it was first approved to restore volume loss in patients with HIV (lipoatrophy).

PLLA is a synthetic polymer made of the same material that comprises Vicryl (absorbable) suture. Its mechanism of action is to cause microscopic nodules of multinucleated giant cells in the subcutaneous tissues (ie, the so-called foreign body reaction). It is subsequently degraded over time by macrophages into lactic acid, then reduced to glucose and carbon dioxide. While the product does generate a foreign body reaction and subsequent inflammation within the body, it is a well-established material that is deemed safe and has excellent long-term efficacy.

Soon after the injection, patients should expect an immediate increase in volume within the face; however, this is only due to the volume of the diluent used to reconstitute the vial of PLLA. These immediate effects are short lived and will gradually disappear over the following few days due to the absorption of the fluid. Over the following weeks, PLLA stimulates the host's own collagen synthesis, leading to the deposition of new collagen in the areas injected. The new collagen produced is volumized in a progressive manner over time. PLLA usually dissolves after 12 to 18 months.

The main indications of PLLA are shallow to deep nasolabial folds, the midface, prejowl folds, and temporal areas. By contrast, there are several areas that the manufacturer recommends avoiding, including the forehead, glabella, crow's feet, hands, neck, and perioral areas such as the lips, oral commissures, and perioral wrinkles.

There have also been reports of delayed-onset nodules and papules forming with PLLA. If you choose any treatment with PLLA, be sure to notify your doctors days in advance because the product will need to be adequately mixed 24 to 72 hours prior to your appointment to minimize any chance of nodule formation. In addition, patients with any history of autoimmune disease should avoid PLLA.

CaHA

Radiesse is a brand of CaHA commonly used for deeper facial wrinkles or defects to restore lost volume.[6] It is composed of 70% aqueous sodium carboxymethyl cellulose gel carrier and 30% synthetic calcium hydroxylapatite microspheres. The nice thing about this product is that it is nonanimal; rather it is derived from *synthetic* sources that are commonly found in bone (ie, HA). Therefore, there is a low risk for allergic reaction, and it is less likely to cause a foreign body reaction.

When deposited in contact with human tissue, CaHA provides immediate soft tissue augmentation due to its gel carrier component. Later on, the carrier gel is gradually absorbed, and CaHA particles induce a histiocytic and fibroblastic response, resulting in the production of new collagen. It is important to note that this material is always injected into deeper planes because superficial injections may cause the material to be visible.

PDO threads

PDO threads are actually spherical, medical-grade threads that are similar in composition to sutures. However, results have shown that when implanted under the skin, PDO threads can lead to collagen formation.[7] In fact, their use has also been associated with hair regrowth.

PDO threads generally dissolve in about 6 to 9 months, but results are expected to last about 1 year because they leave behind new collagen formation. The mode of action is similar to that of PLLA; upon injection, a foreign body reaction leads to an accumulation of infiltrating immune cells that then encapsulate the material. This results in new collagen formation, which helps build volume in the area until the product is fully resorbed 9 months later. PDO threads have also been shown to improve new blood flow (angiogenesis). Like other fillers (Radiesse and Sculptra), PDO threads can be blended with liquid-PRF for added benefits (Figs 9 and 10).

Once again, patients with any history of autoimmune disease should not use PDO threads. However, in patients with healthy immune function, PDO threads are noninvasive and carry very low risk of scarring, bruising, bleeding, or other more serious complications. In rare cases, patients may experience irritation, infection, or visibility of the threads under their skin.

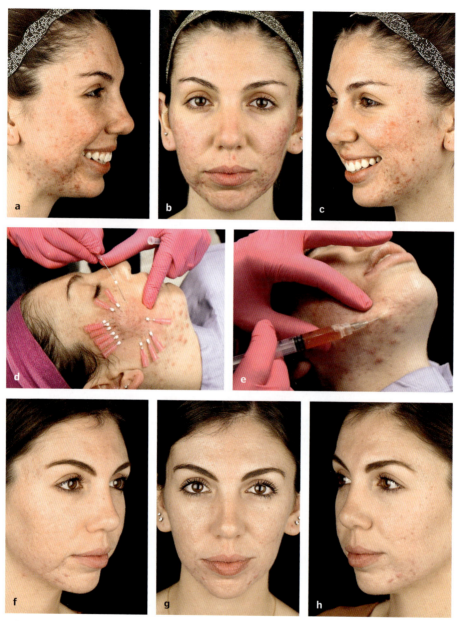

FIG 9 *(a to c)* An 18-year-old woman presented with severe facial acne. First-stage treatment included microneedling with PRF to destroy the active infection. *(d and e)* Second-stage treatment included PDO threads to build collagen and improve the acne scarring. *(f to h)* One year posttreatment. Notice the excellent healing outcomes and facial harmony.

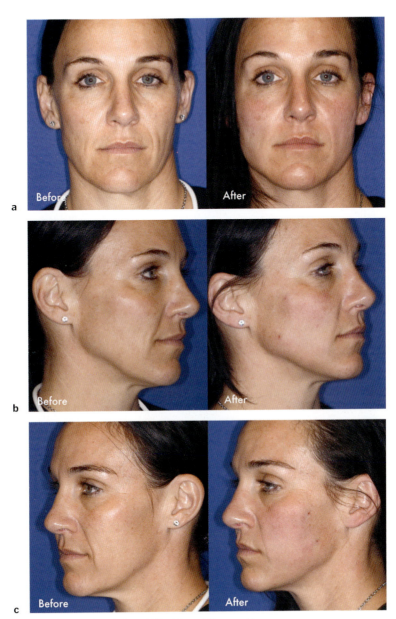

FIG 10 *(a to c)* PDO thread lift of the midface and jaw.

Potential Complications with Fillers

One of the downsides of using facial fillers is their potential risk for complications.[8] Generally speaking, these can be categorized as either mild or serious. Vascular complications are one of the more dangerous complications particularly noted with HA fillers (because they attract water and thus expand). While most fillers may lead to some form of pain and tenderness, bruising, erythema (redness), and swelling at the injection site, more serious complications include allergic reactions, formation of granulomatous tissue, infections, and vascular events such as arterial embolization lead to skin necrosis or blindness.

Early-onset complications

- Edema, pain, erythema, and itching
- Non-inflammatory nodules and contour irregularities
- Tyndall effect/discoloration
- Hypersensitivity reaction
- Vascular event
- Foreign body granulomas

Vascular events

There are a number of issues that may cause a vascular event:

- Compression of a vessel by excessive swelling posttreatment
- Direct intravascular injection leading to embolism or occlusion of the vessel

The danger areas include the glabella and nose, including the tip and alar triangle (Figs 11 and 12). The most serious complication related to vascular occlusion is blindness or visual impairment caused by occlusion of the central retinal artery or one of its branches (Fig 13). Injection sites that are considered danger zones must therefore be avoided to prevent such complications.

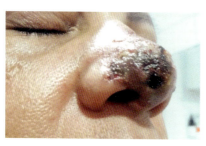

FIG 11 Vascular occlusion of the nasal tip after use of an HA filler. (Reprinted with permission from Garg and Rossi.[9])

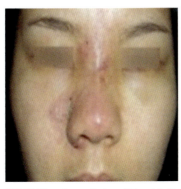
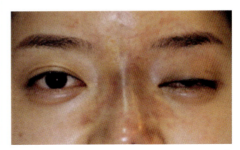

FIG 12 Vascular occlusion of the glabella and nasal region after use of an HA filler. (Reprinted with permission from Kim et al.[10])

FIG 13 Vascular occlusion of the retinal artery leading to visual complications after use of an HA filler. (Reprinted with permission from Myung et al.[11])

References

1. Davis JI, Senghas A, Brandt F, Ochsner KN. The effects of BOTOX injections on emotional experience. Emotion 2010;10:433–440.
2. Satriyasa BK. Botulinum toxin (Botox) A for reducing the appearance of facial wrinkles: A literature review of clinical use and pharmacological aspect. Clin Cosmet Investig Dermatol 2019;12:223–228.
3. Mess SA. Lower face rejuvenation with injections: Botox, Juvederm, and Kybella for marionette lines and jowls. Plast Reconstr Surg Glob Open 2017;5:e1551.
4. Monheit G, Grimes PE, Hardas B, Lin V, Murphy DK. Juvederm Vollure XC is safe and effective for correcting nasolabial folds: Results from a randomized controlled study. SKIN J Cutan Med 2017;1(suppl 3.1):S77.
5. Lam SM, Azizzadeh B, Graivier M. Injectable poly-L-lactic acid (Sculptra): Technical considerations in soft-tissue contouring. Plast Reconstr Surg 2006;118(3 suppl):55S–63S.
6. Jansen DA, Graivier MH. Evaluation of a calcium hydroxylapatite-based implant (Radiesse) for facial soft-tissue augmentation. Plast Reconstr Surg 2006;118(3 suppl):22S–30S.
7. Ali YH. Two years' outcome of thread lifting with absorbable barbed PDO threads: Innovative score for objective and subjective assessment. J Cosmet Laser Ther 2018;20:41–49.
8. Kim D-W, Yoon E-S, Ji Y-H, Park S-H, Lee B-I, Dhong E-S. Vascular complications of hyaluronic acid fillers and the role of hyaluronidase in management. J Plast Reconstr Aesthet Surg 2011;64:1590–1595.
9. Garg AK, Rossi R Jr. Dermal Fillers for Dental Professionals. Chicago: Quintessence, 2021.
10. Kim JH, Ahn DK, Jeong HS, Suh IS. Treatment algorithm of complications after filler injection: Based on wound healing process. J Korean Med Sci 2014;29(suppl 3):S176–S182.
11. Myung Y, Yim S, Jeong JH, et al. The classification and prognosis of periocular complications related to blindness following cosmetic filler injection. Plast Reconstr Surg 2017;140:61–64.

Chapter 9

Bio-Lift and Bio-CARE Protocols

This chapter presents our signature treatments at CARE Esthetics that combine various PRF and laser therapy protocols. These protocols are exclusive to CARE Esthetics and the most frequently performed procedures within our offices.

While all CARE Esthetic providers are trained and certified to offer a multitude of facial esthetic procedures including Botox, PDO threads, and fillers, the main focus at CARE Esthetics is our commitment to a more natural approach that favors better long-term health and maintenance of skin tissues. Thus, all CARE Esthetics providers abide by the following mission statement and undergo yearly education requirements.

> **Mission statement**
>
> *Leading experts in natural esthetic medicine*
> The Center for Advanced Rejuvenation and Esthetics (CARE) is committed to improving the field of facial esthetics by offering more natural approaches and regenerative procedures in facial esthetics. Under the direction of numerous international clinical experts in facial esthetics consisting of leading researchers in platelet concentrates (PRF) and laser therapy, a series of natural regenerative approaches and therapies are performed at CARE Esthetics to obtain beautiful and natural-looking esthetic outcomes.
>
> *Our philosophy: Natural beauty*
> We have a different philosophy in reversing facial aging. At CARE Esthetics, we are proud to use natural regenerative approaches with lasers and PRF without having to utilize unnecessary chemicals or "filling" materials.

Over the past years, we have pioneered and collected data on thousands of cases to determine the most effective ways to regenerate facial tissues using all-natural approaches. These are divided into two main signature treatments: *(1)* the Bio-Lift protocol using an all-natural biomaterial derived from whole blood (PRF therapy), and *(2)* the Bio-CARE protocol combining the original Bio-Lift therapy with laser therapy. **Together, these offer the most advanced, all-natural regenerative strategies available today.**

Signature Treatments

Bio-Lift

The Bio-PRF Lift (or Bio-Lift for short) was developed to establish a multi-step approach using various PRF modalities to unleash and maximize the natural potent bioactivity and regenerative capacity of the human body by using specific protocols.

These protocols, developed in 2017, focus exclusively on PRF in a 100% all-natural approach.

Treatment protocol

The Bio-Lift maximizes the regenerative potential of facial tissues by combining three of our most favored patient treatments backed my medical science:

1. Standard microneedling with PRF (see chapter 6)
2. Bio-PRF injections
3. Natural facial fillers (longer-lasting use of the Bio-Filler technology to treat facial deficiencies)

Therefore, the goal of Bio-Lift therapy is not only to address underlying problems in volume loss with the Bio-Filler (longer-lasting treatment for volume loss) but also to maximize the regenerative potential of the body using PRF. These procedures typically last about 45 minutes, during which time your blood is drawn, centrifuged using a Bio-PRF device, and reintroduced into your facial tissues in concentrated modalities. Figures 1 and 2 demonstrate some case examples.

> CARE Esthetics centers were the first in the world to introduce Bio-Lift protocols to facial esthetics.

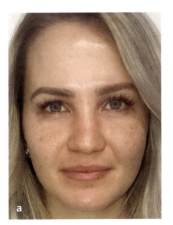
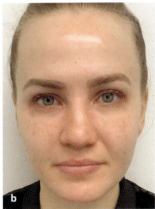

FIG 1 *(a and b)* Note that many young women will begin these therapies in their late 20s and early 30s, not necessarily to improve wrinkles but to maintain or improve long-term skin health and to prevent and minimize facial aging. Notice the obvious glow and improvements in her skin tone simply from one Bio-Lift treatment.

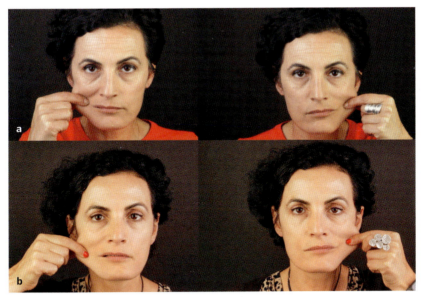

FIG 2 In middle-aged individuals, skin laxity begins to play a factor in skin aging. We routinely ask patients to do the pull test (where they pull on their cheeks) in order to see how loose the skin is. *(a and b)* Following a series of three Bio-Lift protocols each 1 month apart, this woman had noticeable improvements in her skin tone (note the glow-like appearance), improvements in her fine lines and wrinkles, and she also experienced tightening of her skin.

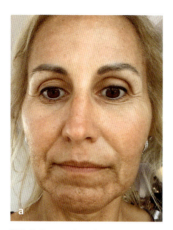 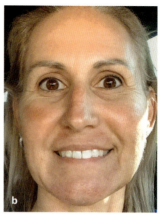

FIG 3 Remember this patient from chapter 6? *(a and b)* In her case, the Bio-Filler was used to add volume in various areas she had lost it (her cheeks, temples, and chin). She was treated three times each 1 month apart with the full Bio-CARE protocol, which is a series of five all-natural steps.

Bio-CARE

As highlighted in chapter 7, the use of lasers in the field of facial esthetics offers a wide range of new and exciting possibilities and means to further enhance facial rejuvenation. For these reasons, in 2019 the Bio-CARE protocol was established by bringing together PRF experts with many laser therapy experts in facial esthetics. Because both therapies are all-natural, the goal was to develop the most potent all-natural regenerative treatment in facial esthetics by combining them. As discussed in chapter 7, laser therapy is able to reactivate dormant fibroblasts to recreate lost collagen. The additional use of PRF, a source of growth factors and stimulating agents, is then able to supplement laser therapy with the building blocks needed for enhanced regeneration. Simply put by one of our CARE Esthetics practitioners, **the laser first activates the fibroblasts to produce more collagen, and the PRF provides the nutrients.** It's just like adding gasoline (PRF) to the fire (laser therapy).

In any event, the Bio-CARE protocol makes up the majority of the treatments we do at CARE Esthetics and was developed for patients who don't want chemical additives in their body but prefer an all-natural approach. The Bio-CARE protocol is as all-natural and as potent as they come, combining the advantages of laser and PRF treatments for maximum facial rejuvenation.

Treatment protocol

The full Bio-CARE protocol is a series of five all-natural steps in a 75-minute procedure (Fig 3):

Step 1: Stimulate collagen production using SmoothLase laser therapy
- SmoothLase is one of the signature treatments of the Fotona laser system, featuring the ability to regenerate and stimulate collagen from the inside of the mouth.
- This therapy precisely targets the nasolabial folds and marionette lines from inside the mouth.

Step 2: Laser peel
- A laser peel is the procedure most commonly desired by celebrities and actors to improve skin turnover and regeneration. It removes a thin layer of the epidermis, giving the skin a freshened look while removing some fine lines and wrinkles.

Step 3: Microneedling with PRF
- Microneedling with PRF enhances facial skin rejuvenation. The goal here is to deliver all the concentrated growth factors found in PRF into the skin to replenish it and give it the ability to heal itself and to produce more collagen to minimize fine lines and wrinkles.

Step 4: Customized treatment plan using Bio-Filler
- Bio-Filler technology was launched as a 100% all-natural way to use PRF as a biologic filler (Bio-Filler). Thus, every person receives a custom treatment plan that aims to fill any volume loss that has occurred over time.

Step 5: Complimentary removal of moles, veins, and age spots
- Each patient receives a personalized treatment plan using 100% natural approaches.

Results obtained using the Bio-CARE protocol

Figures 4 to 10 showcase the results possible when laser therapy is combined with PRF in the Bio-CARE protocol. These are patients just like you who have benefited tremendously from these all-natural procedures.

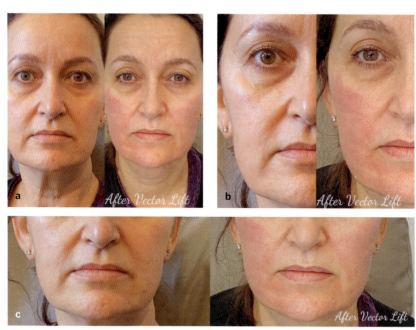

FIG 4 *(a to c)* Note here the effects of laser therapy immediately after treatment. One of the nice things about using lasers is the ability to create and tighten skin using facial "vectors" to lift tissues in a similar way as PDO threads but done entirely naturally. The after photographs are taken directly after the 1-hour procedure. Note these lifted effects seen immediately after treatment.

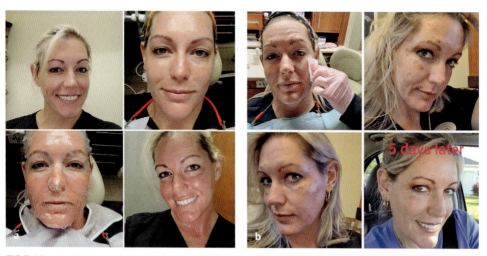

FIG 5 Many patients wonder what a typical posttherapy session will entail. *(a)* These images show one patient following her first Bio-CARE protocol where she had several age spots removed. Most commonly patients will be red for 48 to 72 hours following the laser peel. Microneedling with PRF helps shorten the recovery time because of the growth factors, and it also further improves the results. *(b)* The age spots that were removed will typically be red for roughly 5 days, and scabs will then fall off. It's very typical for patients to send us selfies reporting their progress, so please feel free to do so and to share your experiences on social media!

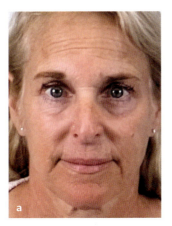
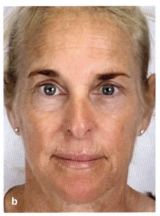

FIG 6 *(a and b)* Before and after photographs following a series of three Bio-CARE treatments. Note the decreases in fine lines and wrinkles and the effects on her nasolabial folds, which were her main concerns. This was achieved all-naturally using the Bio-CARE protocol.

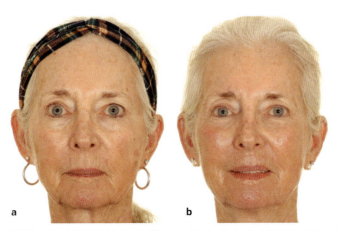

FIG 7 *(a and b)* Meet Nancy, a 72-year-old who looks just fabulous! Hear what she has to say about her experience with the Bio-CARE protocol and how the therapy has helped her reach what she states is "a better version of myself!"

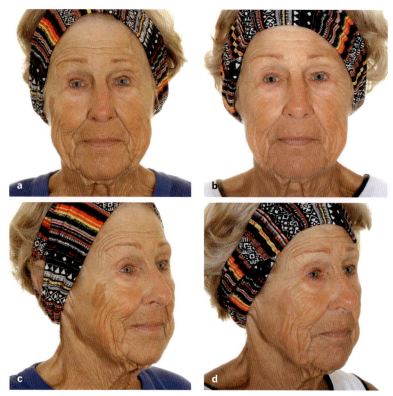

FIG 8 Remember this patient from chapter 2? *(a to d)* She has now gone through her third Bio-CARE treatment, and while we can see marked improvements in her skin, there is still a need for additional regeneration. This highlights that *(1)* skin damage from the sun is far worse than anything else and is always more complex to treat, requiring more therapies—so definitely wear sunscreen if you're in the sun frequently! And *(2)* it is better to start these therapies earlier rather than later. The longer you wait, the harder it is to fully benefit from treatment.

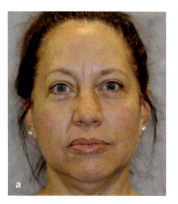
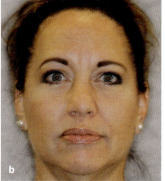

FIG 9 Ideally, we want to start full Bio-CARE protocols when patients are in their early to mid-40s to be able to maintain the esthetic results in the long term. *(a and b)* Take a look at the before and after photographs of this patient after only two treatments.

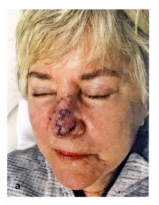
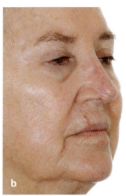
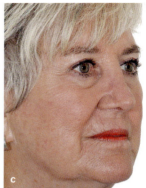
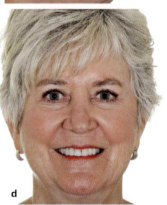

FIG 10 Meet Kathleen. She underwent Mohs surgery for skin cancer removal, which resulted in her surgeon needing to create skin flaps to cover the surgical sites *(a)*. This left Kathleen with many visible scars on her nose, with certain areas of her nose elevated *(b)*. Her case was treated with a series of precise laser therapy protocols and microneedling with PRF to treat her scars. *(c and d)* Today you can hardly tell that Kathleen had anything done in the area at all. After we built her confidence by treating her scars, we then performed two Bio-CARE treatments to lift her skin and decrease her jowls. Hear what she has to say in this video!

Free Consultations and Personalized Treatment Plans

One of the benefits of CARE Esthetics is that all centers provide free consultations. We look forward to listening to your individual goals and fully addressing your esthetic questions. Every individual will have the opportunity to personally meet with our team to review and establish a personalized treatment plan. Call us anytime to schedule your complimentary consultation and to learn more about your options using completely natural and chemical-free approaches!

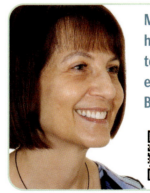

Meet Aleene and hear what she has to say about her experience with the Bio-CARE protocol!

Chapter 10

Cosmeceuticals and Skin Care

Skin care products are a multibillion dollar industry (Fig 1). Billions of dollars go into making them, selling them, and convincing people to use them. Let's be honest: There are *a lot* of products on the market and *a lot* of celebrity endorsements. Because skin care goes *on top* of your body and not into it like PRF, no strict medical testing is required by the US Food and Drug Administration (FDA).

And that's a big problem in the industry. Unlike the other protocols explained in this book that are all heavily researched and regulated by the FDA, many skin care products reference pseudoscience to gain credibility in the hope of differentiating themselves from competitors. It is clear that while some do have beneficial effects, a better understanding of cosmeceuticals as a whole is needed. Let's begin with the basics.

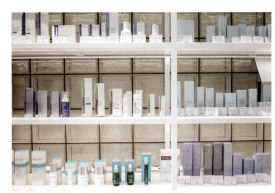

FIG 1 Skin care is big business, which is why there are so many products available.

The Basics

An ideal cosmeceutical product should have the following characteristics:

- Show immediate effect
- Show long-lasting effect
- Carry a low or no side-effect profile
- Be inexpensive
- Treat a wide variety of skin conditions

However, the reality is that most skin care products only fulfill a few of these criteria.

It is also noteworthy that application matters just as much as content when it comes to skin care, because various biomolecules found in skin require different depths of penetration. For instance, vitamin C helps fibroblasts produce collagen. Fibroblasts reside at greater depths within the skin than do epithelial cells. Skin care products that contain vitamin C therefore require an ability for this molecule to penetrate and be delivered to deeper layers of the skin that host fibroblasts. It's not as simple as applying vitamin C on the skin. There is much to regulate, including delivery systems, acidity, stability, pH of delivery, pH when active, and ability to take effect on skin cells. All that is to say, it would be quite impossible for someone to create a new skin care line overnight.

Sunscreen, as another example, should be applied topically at the outermost layer of skin to prevent UV rays from penetrating the skin at all. Thus, the delivery systems for sunscreens and vitamin C are completely different, and therefore these products should not be compounded together. This is one of the main reasons why high-quality skin care products come with a series of topical creams to apply, each targeting different depths of penetration and each being designed with different delivery systems depending on their target skin layer. This will be covered in greater detail later in this chapter.

Remember, too, that skin care products that are improperly made can cause some adverse side effects, such as the irritation often experienced with low-quality retinols. Thus, it is always best to err on the side of caution and to use cosmeceuticals recommended for medical purposes from medical providers, not endorsed by celebrities.

Some myths regarding cosmeceuticals

1. **The more expensive the cream, the better.** This is often not the case, and celebrity endorsements can often cloud reality and perception.
2. **Moisturizers remove wrinkles**. No, they simply reduce their appearance primarily through increased skin hydration. To remove or eliminate wrinkles, regenerative therapies are needed, and a variety of rejuvenating procedures like PRF or laser therapy are highlighted in previous chapters of this book.

3. **Natural automatically means safe and effective.** Some of the most irritant and allergenic products are "natural" extracts of plants. Furthermore, plant extracts require even less testing by the FDA to be approved for commercial sale, despite the fact that some are the most toxic products on the market, even when compared with their synthetically derived relatives.
4. **Topical application of skin care has the same effect as oral supplementation through pills.** This is most certainly not true. Always remember that topical delivery to an area allows for a greater concentration within that targeted tissue and thus better activity. Vitamin E is the classic example—it is very effective when applied on skin but has little impact when taken orally in pill form.
5. **Cosmeceuticals must penetrate the skin barrier to work.** This is important for some products, but others, such as products that block the sun, are in fact better suited overlaying the skin. Thus, different delivery modalities and delivery systems are required depending on the task and benefit of each cosmeceutical.

> For detailed information on classes of cosmeceuticals and their specific applications, scan this QR code.

Skin Care Terms to Know

There is a lot of terminology and technicality in the cosmeceutical industry. To help you wade through it all, here we provide some common terminology from the industry followed by short definitions, almost like a dictionary for skin care.

Alpha hydroxy acids (AHAs): AHAs include glycolic acid, lactic acid, and malic acid. They are primarily used in exfoliating agents, but at higher concentrations they can peel the skin.

Antioxidants: Products that prevent or inhibit the oxidation of other molecules (by free radicals) and can protect cells from the damaging effects of oxidation. This effect is particularly useful with sun damage, pollutions, smoking, etc. Antioxidants in these examples prevent skin damage, thus allowing for maintenance of damage-free skin barriers.

Botanicals: Plant extracts often found in skin care products. They do not require extensive testing and therefore are often cheaper, but sometimes more irritant to the skin.

Cosmeceuticals: Products that are neither pure cosmetics nor drugs but have elements of both.

Emollients: Products with a lipid content that produce a layer on the skin, reducing transepidermal water loss and thereby soothing and hydrating the skin.

Hydroquinone: Used to even out skin tone. It is an inhibitor of melanin production often used in depigmentation creams to lighten the skin. Very commonly used in Asian culture where it is more "trendy" to have whiter skin tones.

Melasma: A condition causing hyperpigmentation on the face of women, often associated with pregnancy and/or dysregulation of hormones such as estrogens (both endogenous and exogenous).

Peptides: Short chains of amino acid sequences. There are three types of peptides used by the cosmeceutical industry: signal peptides, carrier peptides, and neurotransmitter inhibitor peptides. They often work by taking action in the skin and are most commonly produced synthetically.

Retinoids: A large family of vitamin A (retinol) analogs derived from beta carotene. Retinoids act by turning over skin cells at a faster rate by activating the nuclear retinoid receptors. Retinols and their family are discussed at length later in this chapter because they are some of the most studied cosmeceutical compounds.

Rosacea: A skin condition causing redness in which there is telangiectasia of blood and lymph vessels.

Sunscreens: Creams or compounds that either physically reflect light and have a broad spectrum of action (such as titanium dioxide or zinc oxide) or chemically absorb UV light and re-emit it as heat (such as para-aminobenzoic acid, benzophenones, and cinnamates).

Conditions Treated by Cosmeceuticals

Photodamage

As discussed in chapter 2, photodamage caused by UV rays is one of the fastest ways to speed facial aging (recall that photo of the truck driver). A number of changes to the skin occur because of prolonged exposure to UV rays, such as atrophy, telangiectasia, fine and deep wrinkles, yellowing (solar elastosis), and dyspigmentation.

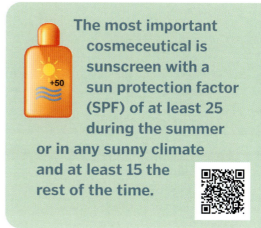

The most important cosmeceutical is sunscreen with a sun protection factor (SPF) of at least 25 during the summer or in any sunny climate and at least 15 the rest of the time.

Hyperpigmentation

Hyperpigmentation is a result of sun exposure, overheating of melanocytes, or hormonal changes (for example, melasma). Pigmented lesions may be superficial or deep. In both cases, the excess melanin is contained within epidermal melanocytes and can be treated by topical cosmeceuticals.

Deep hyperpigmentation is usually due to postinflammatory changes, and the excess melanin is often contained in macrophages deeper in the dermis where it is difficult for topical agents to exert an effect. The most effective cosmeceutical for hyperpigmentation is hydroquinone, which works by inhibiting the conversion of tyrosine to melanin. Typically, this is prescribed in a 4% concentration. Hyperpigmentation is often treated with a combination of laser therapy and cosmeceuticals.

Facial redness

Facial redness may be a caused by a variety of factors (many of which are genetic) ranging from excessive heat to exercise, alcohol, spicy food, and stress. Patients with rosacea are often more sensitive and intolerant of many skin care products. In advising on skin care products, it may even be necessary to use cheaper products with fewer ingredients, as these are less likely to irritate the skin.

For definite rosacea, the most effective topical products are metronidazole (Rozex Cream) and azelaic acid (Finacea Cream). It is important to avoid potent topical steroids, which lead to temporary relief followed by even worse rebound.

Wrinkles

Wrinkles and facial aging are caused primarily by extrinsic factors such as photodamage. Intrinsic/genetic factors contribute only about 10% of the time.

The #1 cosmeceutical for treatment of wrinkles is retinoids at various concentrations. Noteworthy, however, is that these should never be utilized at the same time as common regenerative therapies such as lasers, because the combination will certainly overirritate the skin and could potentially lead to additional redness. It is therefore recommended that retinols are stopped 1 week prior to regenerative treatment and discontinued for 1 month after therapy.

General skin health

Cosmeceuticals may seem trivial, having little effect on aging skin, but in fact, use of cosmeceuticals may very well be the most important recommendation for long-term skin health and beauty. After all, **it is the long-term preventive care that is needed to maintain excellent skin.**

> **The importance of daily skin care and sunscreen use cannot be overstated! Just ask any Hollywood celebrity who looks way younger than his or her actual age.**

Of course, there are so many skin care products available on the market that it may seem overwhelming to patients at first. But with a few simple guidelines, skin care can become an easy habit to keep. We'll show you how.

It is important to remember that skin care products are not necessarily meant to reverse the signs of aging like PRF or laser therapy, but instead, they act to prevent *future* damage/aging. No cosmeceutical product can remove deep lines and wrinkles, but certainly many studies have shown improvements in fine lines using medical-grade cosmeceuticals, especially when used in combination with regenerative therapies. Most studies look at results at 90 days, once again highlighting the fact that small and gradual changes should be expected over time, not overnight miracles.

Posttreatment Skin Care and Its Effect on Aging Skin

This section was written by Geir Håvard Kvalheim, the founder of the skin care line Čuvget, a highly respected Norwegian brand of facial creams and serums developed based on scientific research. It is adapted from the original chapter published in *PRF in Facial Esthetics*.[1] The goal of this section is to provide the science behind why medical-grade cosmeceuticals are more valuable than your over-the-counter variety. Let's go!

Posttreatment Skin Care

Posttreatment skin care is a crucial step aimed at enhancing the clinical results following facial esthetic procedures. In general, skin care products usually only penetrate 8% into the skin. When microneedling is performed, however, penetration can reach up to 80% to 90% depth for up to 72 hours. The application of ideal skin products not only helps to stimulate and regenerate skin cells, improving their collagen synthesis, but may also modulate the inflammatory response posttreatment, thereby significantly reducing patient downtime. This section explores the recent research dedicated to improving skin care and introduces various extracts that are able to promote wound healing. Specifically, Norwegian scientists who spent decades studying the harsh arctic climate discovered that a specific mushroom (chaga) surviving in these northern climates carried potent and powerful antioxidants capable of drastically reducing oxidative damage by as much as 80% within an hour. Following years of research on the topic, these novel extracts have since been formulated within skin care products (Čuvget).

Skin Rejuvenation and Healing

It has been demonstrated that a specific skin care regimen following facial esthetic procedures may reduce the "downtime" required for healing, improve the esthetic results, and ultimately give the patient a better experience. Specific ingredients delivered via topical skin care products can create a synergistic effect with facial esthetic treatments like PRF and laser therapy to maximize rejuvenation while minimizing healing time.

The biologic effects of initiating a potent skin care posttreatment regimen are based on three core steps:

1. Activating immune cells and reducing inflammation caused by controlled damage
2. Stimulating the epidermal rejuvenation processes
3. Enhancing epidermal protection from extrinsic aging factors and improving water retention

Step 1: Activating Immune Cells and Reducing Inflammation

The controlled damage inflicted on the epidermal layer of the skin during facial esthetic procedures triggers a cascade reaction, eventually resulting in skin rejuvenation. Clinical trials have concluded that immediately after treatment of the epidermis, a combination of immune-modulating agents and potent antioxidants results in both a short- and long-term advantage, favoring healing and minimizing downtime post-therapy. PRF can improve regenerative outcomes in the short-term, but topical use of medical-grade cosmeceuticals can extend these results long-term.

Over the past decade, scientists at the University of Tromsø in Norway have developed world-leading competence on biologic properties of arctic extracts. The hypothesis was that because the arctic environment represents one of the harshest and coldest climate conditions on the planet, and because species found in this area have developed extreme protection mechanisms as an adaptation, a better understanding of their biologic behavior could lead to breakthrough research for medical applications. In 2014, after investigating thousands of extracts, the research team discovered that a specific extract concentrated from a mushroom called *chaga* (trademarked Čaga) led to potent wound-healing properties. This extract is extremely useful in improving the potency of cosmeceuticals.

Arctic Čaga extract

Arctic Čaga extract has its origin from a rare species of parasitic fungus growing on the bark of genus *Betula* trees in the northern parts of the world. It has a rich background in folk medicine as tinctures and tea to aid the immune system and suppress infections.

The Arctic Čaga extract is produced from the conk (shelf) of wild Nordic chaga fungus. It contains a rich composition of bioactive compounds including polysaccharides, beta-glucans, and polyphenols that in skin care formulations are designed to reduce the "downtime" after invasive esthetic treatments, because they contain potent levels of antioxidants. In fact, ancient medicine from the Norwegian indigenous people have called it the "mushroom of immortality" and the "diamond of the forest." Various preparations of Čaga, including Čaga tea, have been used in the past to treat complicated diseases and immune disorders.

Over the years, scientific focus has been directed toward this unique extract and its potential health benefits and/or application for new treatments in the fight against various diseases. The skin care company Čuvget has since adopted its formulation in its vitamin ampoules.

Antioxidant properties

Research conducted by Fenola demonstrated that the Arctic Čaga extract scored extremely high in its antioxidant analysis scores (ScandiDerma, unpublished research, 2016). The Arctic Čaga extract exhibits a very potent antioxidative effect on a skin keratocyte model, and several studies have reported a dramatic reduction of oxidative damage (up to 80% observed within 60 minutes).

Epidermal volume

The Čuvget Instant Vitamin Ampoules have been shown to increase the epidermal volume by 50% compared to controls (skin equivalents not treated with Instant Vitamin Ampoules). The skin surface also showed a significantly smoother appearance with an even distribution of skin cells

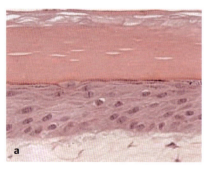 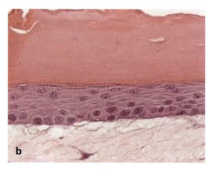

FIG 2 *(a and b)* Note the 50% increase in epidermal volume with Čuvget Instant Vitamin Ampoules after 1 week of treatment, which clinically translates to a reduction in fine lines and wrinkles. (Study performed by ScandiDerma in collaboration with Epistem Ltd, unpublished.)

as a result of an improved epidermal performance. Histologic evaluation also demonstrated a significantly larger surface volume compared to controls (Fig 2).

Immunomodulating properties

Another important aspect following any facial esthetic treatment is the management of inflammation after the procedure. Therefore, products and ingredients developed to modulate the immune system following therapy may lead to faster healing. The Arctic Čaga extract contains a rich and natural concentration of beta-glucans, with the key target of activating the Langerhans (immune) cells. Langerhans cells are the modulators of the skin because they serve as the control center managing crucial biologic processes. These cells are well known as protective cells ("magistrate cells"), residing in the upper layers of the skin, and they protect against both invading microorganisms and other skin damage. Beta-glucans have vast documentation[2,3] and have been shown to do the following:

Čuvget also includes significant epidermal antioxidants. To learn more, scan this QR code.

- Increase renewal of skin cells (rejuvenation)
- Stimulate the production of collagen and other growth factors of the skin
- Repair skin cells damaged by UV rays
- Optimize the normal processes of human skin via the Langerhans cells

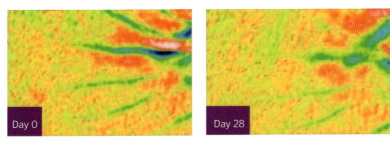

FIG 3 Thirty-two volunteers between 40 and 60 years old with signs of photoaged skin were given the active formula of 1.5% Lingostem on one half of the face and one forearm, while a placebo was used on the other half of the face and the other forearm. Volunteers applied the extract twice daily for 28 days. Note the repairing effect of the cream on eye contour wrinkles at 28 days.

Step 2: Stimulating Epidermal Rejuvenation

Clinical studies have demonstrated that treating the skin with a complex of collagen-inducing therapies and protective ingredients will enhance the effects of facial rejuvenation procedures. Therefore, a stimulating serum is the basis of many esthetic creams developed to target fibroblast activity and induce collagen synthesis. Several active ingredients are carefully formulated to stimulate epidermal rejuvenation, as highlighted below.

Lingonberry stem cell extract—Lingostem

Arctic berries have been known to contain a high concentration of polyphenols that protect cells from reactive oxygen species (ROS).[4] A research project in collaboration with the University of Tromsø, the Norwegian Institute of Bioeconomy Research, and the Technical Research Centre of Finland concluded that arctic lingonberry leaves contain potent antioxidant properties. Stem cell extract is obtained from lingonberry, which is rich in polyphenols and traditionally used by the indigenous people of the north for its antioxidant healing properties. Lingostem is a formulation of lingonberry stem cells designed to prevent and reverse photoaging, mimicking one of nature's solutions to fight damaging effects of solar radiation in plants. Clinical studies with the same concentration as applied in the Čuvget Stimulating Serum show a 37% reduction in the number of wrinkles after 28 days of use (Fig 3).

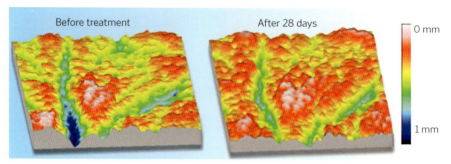

FIG 4 After only 1 month, SYN-TC showed significant improvement in skin smoothness (+9.1%). The effect was further pronounced after 2 months (+12.2%).

Beta-Glucan M

Beta-Glucan M, also called *sodium carboxymethyl beta-glucan*, is known to soothe irritated skin, support the skin's own antioxidant activity, protect the skin from environmental damage, and help the skin retain moisture. In one study, the application of a placebo emulsion counteracted the photoaging process of the skin slightly. The incorporation of only 0.04% Beta-Glucan M into the same emulsion led to a 30% improvement in skin firmness on day 14 and 80% improvement in skin firmness on day 28. In the end, Beta-Glucan M performed 60% better than the placebo and 100% better than the untreated area at day 28 (ScandiDerma, unpublished research, 2016).

Peptides—SYN-TC

Synthetic tripeptide and tetrapeptide (eg, SYN-TC) are other key ingredients added to facial care products due to their ability to significantly increase the amount of stable and homogenous collagen facilitating smooth skin. Clinical studies of SYN-TC with the same concentration as applied in the Čuvget Stimulating Serum showed a significant improvement of skin smoothness and firmness after 28 days of use (ScandiDerma, unpublished research, 2016). 3D imaging confirmed significant reduction of visible signs of aging (Fig 4).

Step 3: Multilayer Protection and Rejuvenation

Invasive treatments trigger rejuvenation but also expose the skin to damaging external environmental effects. A multilayer protection giving the epidermis an optimal layer against external exposure is therefore needed. The Čuvget Protective Day Cream is designed to immediately aid the various epidermal layers through combining UVA and UVB protection with potent ingredients that improve the performance of cell membranes and scavenging ROS.

Omega-3—Omegatri

Cell membranes are composed of phospholipids and other membrane lipids, with membrane proteins interspersed. Cell membranes with an optimal fatty acid composition including an appropriate amount of omega-3 will help keep the appropriate flexibility and hydration of the tissue, and, for skin cells, thus keep the skin soft and protect against dryness. The moisturizing effects of omega-3 are therefore essential. Recent studies have shown that a diet low in essential fatty acids (which applies to about 99% of the US population) can lead to dry skin and premature wrinkles. Boosting the intake of fatty acids will improve smoothness and radiance of the skin. To keep skin cells moist and strong, sufficient intake of omega-3 is strongly recommended.

Omega-3's effects on skin include the stimulation of tissue repair[5] (Fig 5) and the enhancement of collagen production.[6] The variety of positive effects of omega-3 will altogether help keep the skin healthy and strong, enabling it to withstand stress caused by external and internal factors. The preventive and reparative effects of omega-3 give reason for recommending omega-3 cream for relaxing and repairing skin that is damaged.[7]

Typically, omega-3 is delivered via encapsulation in facial creams. Omegatri technology is an award-winning encapsulation technique developed to promote epidermal uptake and stabilize the omega-3 oils to ensure optimal performance and stability.

Arnica

Another important component is arnica. It exerts anti-inflammatory effects by inhibiting prostaglandin production. A clinical study revealed that twice-

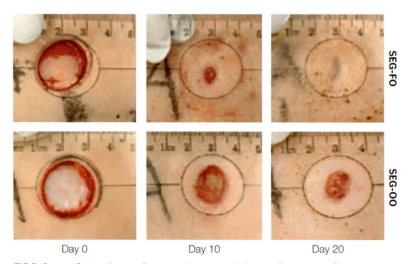

FIG 5 Omega-3 stimulates collagen production and is known for its anti-inflammatory properties. Several studies show how polyunsaturated fatty acids are able to significantly improve skin healing within 20 days. (Reprinted with permission from Shingel et al.[5])

daily application of an arnica-containing gel for 3 to 6 weeks to 79 patients suffering from knee osteoarthritis significantly reduced joint pain in most of the cases, and the product was well tolerated in 87% of the cases.[8] Therefore, arnica extract is highly recommended in formulations of cosmetic products for sensitive and/or irritated skin and to stimulate general blood circulation.

Arctic Čaga extract—UV protection

Chronic exposure of the skin to UV radiation is known to induce a multitude of harmful effects such as skin thickening, wrinkle formation, inflammation, and even carcinogenesis. These effects have been shown to arise from a continuous oxidative stress state from excessive generation of ROS from exposure to UV radiation, which ultimately leads to cell apoptosis (cell death) events and the breakdown of collagen and thus to the aforementioned undesired morphologic changes in the skin.

Chaga extracts contain a considerable amount of melanin-type polyphenolic pigment compounds that offer a good amount of UV-scattering and UV-absorbing qualities in addition to the power to scavenge free radicals after exposure to UV radiation. These benefits have been shown through in

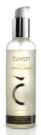 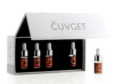 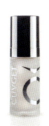 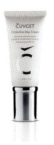 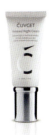

| Exfoliating Foaming Cleanser | Instant Vitamin Ampoules | Stimulating Serum | Protective Day Cream | Renewal Night Cream |

FIG 6 Čuvget 24-hour protocol.

vivo skin models where Čaga has been demonstrated to have remarkable potential at reducing and almost completely suppressing UV-induced skin thickening and wrinkle formation, when applied topically after repetitive exposure to UV radiation, comparable to that of high-concentration retinol.[9]

Application of Čuvget Skin Care Products

The standard set of post-procedure skin care products includes various products, each designed to help maintain the hydration of skin, modulate the immune response, improve collagen synthesis, and protect against external factors (Fig 6). These effects cannot be performed in an all-in-one formulation because cosmeceuticals require proper delivery and penetrate to different depths to target different skin layers. Čuvget does not contain any parabens, and all ingredients are strictly tested by scientists to ensure their safety. An example of such rigorous testing in medical-grade cosmeceuticals can be found here. ··············>

Step 1: Exfoliating Foaming Cleanser

The Exfoliating Foaming Cleanser is used to cleanse and exfoliate the skin twice per day, in the morning and evening. One pump of the cleanser is massaged in the palm of the hand before applying it to the face, neck, and décolletage (Fig 7). This is an enzymatic cleanser, not an acid, which makes it generally less irritant to the skin. The potent enzymes must be allowed

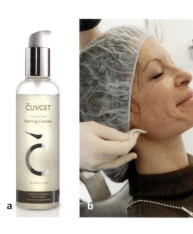

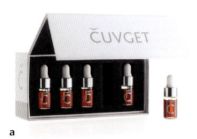
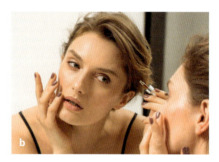

FIG 7 (a) Čuvget Exfoliating Foaming Cleanser. (b) Cleanser being applied to the face.

FIG 8 (a) Čuvget Instant Vitamin Ampoules. (b) A single dropper is applied to all areas of the face and neck.

to work for a 2-minute period before rinsing off the cleanser with water and gently patting the skin dry with a clean towel. The product provides immediate and gentle exfoliation in a pH-friendly formulation for gentle but effective cleansing.

Step 2: Instant Vitamin Ampoules

Immediately after cleansing the skin, a single dropper of the Instant Vitamin Ampoules liquid should be applied on all areas of the face and neck (Fig 8). The Instant Vitamin Ampoules formulation absorbs quickly and targets the deepest layers of the skin, specifically the Langerhans cells with their immunomodulating effect. Instant Vitamin Ampoules also contain a rich cocktail of Arctic Čaga, one of the most potent epidermal antioxidants. Ideally, your CARE Esthetics center will additionally load the Instant Vitamin Ampoules with your own growth factors found in PRF. This allows for your

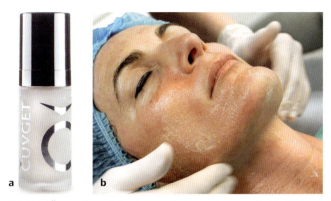

FIG 9 (a) Čuvget Stimulating Serum. (b) Serum being applied to the face.

body's natural healing potential to supplement the ampoules, leading to further improvements in healing and skin rejuvenation.

Step 3: Stimulating Serum

Thereafter, one pump of the Stimulating Serum is applied to the face. Stimulating Serum focuses on total collagen care and maintaining a healthy skin matrix. The product is composed of extracts from stem cells of arctic berries, marine extracts with potent peptides, as well as beta-glucans. While the serum does not penetrate as deeply as the Instant Vitamin Ampoules, the extracts actively target collagen synthesis and increase hydration and cell protection. In combination, these intense ingredients have shown to uniquely reduce the signs of aging. The serum creates an optimal environment and performance of the skin's matrix, leaving the skin surface perfectly smooth and younger looking, with improved radiance and glow (Fig 9).

Step 4: Protective Day/Renewal Night Cream

The final step involves the application of either the Protective Day Cream (in the morning) or the Renewal Night Cream (in the evening). Once again, a single pump is used, and the cream is applied evenly on the skin (Figs 10 and 11).

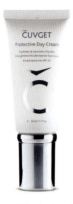

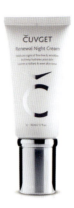

FIG 10 Čuvget Protective Day Cream.

FIG 11 Čuvget Renewal Night Cream.

The Protective Day Cream is the ultimate product against daytime free radical exposure and skin aging. It contains encapsulated retinols, which ensures transdermal delivery. It also contains a unique complex of omega-3 technology and plant-based Arctic Čaga extract and carries an SPF of 37.

The Renewal Night Cream is a unique combination of Arctic plant extracts that focus on stimulating night repair of the skin cells and barrier functions. The cream improves hydration and skin elasticity and reduces the signs of fine lines and wrinkles. The Renewal Night Cream will stimulate skin repair and work against both extrinsic and intrinsic aging to ensure optimal skin rejuvenation.

For details on the key ingredients in the Čuvget line, scan this QR code.

Conclusion

As you can see, the science behind products and their ingredients actually matters. That is why you should always opt for facial cosmeceuticals that have been researched and tested in legitimate scientific laboratories—not the new product endorsed by your favorite celebrity.

References

1. Davies C, Miron RJ (eds). PRF in Facial Esthetics. Chicago: Quintessence, 2020.
2. Arlian LG, Morgan MS, Neal JS. Modulation of cytokine expression in human keratinocytes and fibroblasts by extracts of scabies mites. Am J Trop Med Hyg 2003;69:652–656.
3. Persaud R, Re T. The impact of the skin's innate immunity by cosmetic products applied to the skin and scalp. In: Dayan N, Wertz PW (eds). Innate Immune System of Skin and Oral Mucosa. Hoboken: Wiley, 2011:275–279.
4. Wang SY, Feng R, Bowman L, Penhallegon R, Ding M, Lu Y. Antioxidant activity in lingonberries (*Vaccinium vitis-idaea* L.) and its inhibitory effect on activator protein-1, nuclear factor-KB, and mitogen-activated protein kinases activation. J Agric Food Chem 2005;53:3156–3166.
5. Shingel KI, Faure MP, Azoulay L, Roberge C, Deckelbaum RJ. Solid emulsion gel as a vehicle for delivery of polyunsaturated fatty acids: Implications for tissue repair, dermal angiogenesis and wound healing. J Tissue Eng Regen Med 2008;2:383–393.
6. Hankenson KD, Watkins BA, Schoenlein IA, Allen KGD, Turek JJ. Omega-3 fatty acids enhance ligament fibroblast collagen formation in association with changes in interleukin-6 production. Proc Soc Exp Biol Med 2000;223:88–95.
7. Schwartz S. Lotion sickness: Are your cosmetics making you ill? South China Morning Post. 26 May 2009.
8. Alonso J. Tratado de Fitofármacos y Nutracéuticos. Barcelona: Corpus, 2004:178–182.
9. Joo JI, Kim DH, Yun JW. Extract of Chaga mushroom (*Inonotus obliquus*) stimulates 3T3-L1 adipocyte differentiation. Phytother Res 2010;24:1592–1599.

Chapter 11

The Future of Regenerative Medicine

We are living in some pretty exciting times, with much hope for regenerative medicine to extend both the quality and quantity of life. Some of the regenerative outcomes we see on a daily basis were once considered impossible. Time has allowed for better therapies than ever before, with the newest technologies often reversing lifelong injuries and illnesses. These reversals can be life-changing for patients with Parkinson's or complex knee pain or spinal issues. All of a sudden they can live normally again! This chapter briefly discusses novel regenerative medicine therapies and strategies that will certainly become mainstream in the coming years as more research is gathered.

Extracellular Matrix

The extracellular matrix (ECM) simply refers to the matrix living outside the cell.[1] Certain ECMs are rich in growth factors and have significant wound healing properties; they are able to "feed" the cells appropriate growth hormones and factors to improve their function.[2]

ECMs are therefore popular delivery systems in regenerative therapy. One product that has commonly been used for hair regeneration is ACell's nonsynthetic, fully resorbable device, MatriStem UBM.[3] ACell is processed in a way to remove all living cellular content and mitigation factors that affect potential inflammatory responses (to minimize the foreign body reaction described in chapter 3). The end product contains structures and molecular components like collagen and other proteins (laminin and proteoglycans), all of which are essential during the healing process. ACell has also been shown to favor an environment assisting in minimizing inflammation and potential scar formation.

A second commonly used ECM today is that obtained during amniotic/placental matrix harvesting.[4] Amniotic fluid can easily be collected shortly after birth from the placenta of healthy newborns. Because the placenta is part of the uterine wall of a pregnant woman that surrounds the fetus, it is extremely rich in growth factors, growth hormones, and other nutrients important for healing. These placental tissues are typically discarded during pregnancy, but research labs have been collecting them and intensively studying their regenerative capacities for years.

Research in this field first started with successful treatments of damaged joints, spinal tissues, and complex wounds,[5-7] but amniotic fluid has more recently been utilized in many fields of medicine, including facial esthetics and hair regrowth procedures. Research has shown that amniotic fluid reduces pain at damaged joints, cuts the healing process nearly in half, and also contributes to muscle, tendon, and ligament regeneration. Randomized clinical trials have shown that it has similar regenerative potential to locally harvested stem cells, without the more time-consuming and invasive therapies that locally harvest stem cells from bone marrow or fat deposits.

Stem Cell Harvesting

Today it is possible to harvest your own stem cells in a relatively minimally invasive procedure. These are typically harvested from fat tissue, spun down or digested via various recommended manufacturing protocols, and thereafter utilized for tissue regeneration.[8] The advantage is that autologous stem cells (meaning they are coming from your own body) can be used to facilitate healing without causing a foreign body reaction (because like PRF, they are derived from your own body, so your body will not recognize them as being foreign).

One of the downsides is that stem cell harvesting is quite expensive compared with other regenerative therapies and also typically requires a second surgical/healing site to harvest them. Because of the added cost, time, and secondary potential complications, many clinicians prefer other less invasive regenerative strategies such as combining amniotic fluid with exosomes and PRF. Nevertheless, if more aggressive strategies are required in the case of advanced degeneration, local harvesting of autologous stem cells is a viable option.[9] It does not pose any concern whatsoever to the all-so-precious immune system. Thus, for individuals with a history of allergic responses or hypersensitivities, this is an alternative treatment worth considering, especially for damaged joints.

However, it is not recommended to use stem cells from other sources (like from someone else's body). This can be dangerous. You'll notice that all other biomaterials in this section make absolute certain to remove all living cells from other living donors in order to avoid serious immune-related complications.

> For those looking at stem cell therapy as an option, remember to be certain they are coming from your own body and not someone else's!

Mechanical Transduction and Ultrasonic/Bioelectric Stimulation

Many years ago, basic laboratory experiments determined that by literally stretching cells out on various types of stretchable biomaterials, they would begin to produce more collagen. Thus, the act of mechanically stimulating cells created an entire field within medicine; today many companies focus on some sort of transduction of cells either via mechanical, ultrasonic, or bioelectric means.

Probably the most utilized methods are microfocused or bioelectric stimulation, which are treatments developed to tighten skin by noninvasive/nonsurgical means. These technologies often use heat and ultrasonic wavelengths to improve facial sagging or body contouring. Ultrasound waves can reach and warm the deeper layers of the skin, in which the contraction of collagen begins to occur. The energy is focused at a point below the surface of the skin and concentrated in an area that assists in thermal coagulation to a depth of up to 5 mm in the deeper layers of the skin, without damaging the more superficial layers.[10] This type of therapy is used more frequently for body tightening. Newer research in that space has focused on high-intensity focused ultrasound (HIFU), which was commercialized with increasing popularity.[11] The HIFU is able to produce discrete thermal injury zones delivered to specific areas, leading to better results compared with conventional ultrasound.[11]

Even more novel has been the continued trend to study bioelectric signals. Within the past 3 to 5 years, a team of researchers based in California and Utah have been able to create very specific and short bioelectric wavelength treatments that are geared toward the specific stimulation of single genes. In essence, with a very specific frequency, one can upregulate single genes such as vascular endothelial growth factor (VEGF) or elastin production, for instance.[12] The ability to do so allows for the specific delivery of targeted growth factors in a specific sequence/order at specific time intervals. This patented technology can be used on skin to specifically stimulate the upregulation of elastin followed by collagen and platelet-derived growth factors, all delivered in sequential order. Furthermore, it is possible to bioelectrically stimulate PRF prior to its use. Future research in this field is ongoing and particularly exciting.

Growth Factors, Peptides, and Exosomes

This area of research is probably the fastest growing, safest, and most deserving of considerable attention. Growth factors are small biomolecules found in the body that assist with growth of cells (as the name implies). Years ago, specific growth factors were isolated and fabricated in what is called "recombinant" fashion—which basically means made in a lab to be similar in activity to the real thing.[13] Similarly, many peptides have been added to facial creams and are commonly used to help support facial regeneration. One of the main disadvantages of growth factors and peptides is their relatively short bioactivity (we call this their half-life), which is somewhere between a few minutes to a few hours max. Thus, autologous sources have been more frequently preferred (such as PRF).

One area of research that could bring significant breakthrough is the entire field of exosomes.[14,15] Companies are currently being seeded with

Hear what Matt has to say about getting his knees injected with immunosomes delivered via PRF.

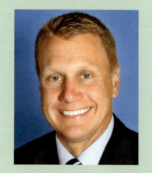

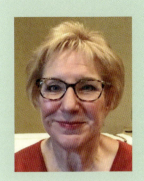

Hear what Linda has to say about her treatments for Parkinson's disease with immunosomes.

hundreds of millions of dollars in research funding to further expand this field. Exosomes, unlike recombinant growth factors and peptides, are small vesicles in which signaling factors are stored and allowed to communicate between cells. The major advantage of exosomes is that they have a much longer activity, on the order of hours to days as opposed to a few minutes, and they are more easily able to penetrate various tissue layers such as the blood-brain barrier (which means they can help heal brain-related injuries such as Parkinson's and multiple sclerosis).[16] Research has now shown that exosomes derived from various sources such as stem cells and amniotic fluid can be utilized for different regenerative purposes and do not cause a negative response to the immune system—some actually help it considerably.

Exosomes that are derived specifically for immune cell function (immunosomes) have already been used for the treatment of complex disorders such as multiple sclerosis and Parkinson's disease. They can be administered intravenously for systemic disorder treatment, and they can target diseased and injured tissues directly. They can also be utilized for the repair of joints when combined with liquid-PRF and delivered locally. In fact, research has shown that exosomes routinely performed better than stem cells from amniotic fluid.[17] In facial esthetics and hair regeneration, exosomes are often combined with liquid-PRF and delivered via microneedling. Their anti-inflammatory response along with their regenerative potential make them ideal for the field of regenerative medicine with much upside in the coming years.

Conclusion

Regenerative medicine is booming, and a number of novel technologies will become available as more research is performed. Always remember the importance of selecting therapies that favor immune cell health and that gauge your own personal experiences with biomaterials. For instance, if you've had negative reactions or allergic reactions to a facial filler, I would avoid implanting other biomaterials such as ECM from various donors and instead favor autologous therapies such as bioelectric stimulation or autologous stem cells. Every person is unique, and it is important to understand that each unique person will respond to implanted biomaterials differently.

References

1. Hay ED. Cell Biology of Extracellular Matrix. Philadelphia: Springer, 2013.
2. Taipale J, Keski-Oja J. Growth factors in the extracellular matrix. FASEB J 1997;11:51–59.
3. Kim JS, Kaminsky AJ, Summitt JB, Thayer WP. New innovations for deep partial-thickness burn treatment with ACell MatriStem Matrix. Adv Wound Care (New Rochelle) 2016;5:546–552.
4. Loukogeorgakis SP, De Coppi P. Concise review: Amniotic fluid stem cells: The known, the unknown, and potential regenerative medicine applications. Stem Cells 2017;35: 1663–1673.
5. Bhattacharya N. Clinical use of amniotic fluid in osteoarthritis: A source of cell therapy. In: Bhattacharya N, Stubblefield P (eds). Regenerative Medicine Using Pregnancy-Specific Biological Substances. London: Springer, 2011:395–403.
6. Friel NA, de Girolamo L, Gomoll AH, Mowry KC, Vines JB, Farr J. Amniotic fluid, cells, and membrane application. Oper Tech Sports Med 2017;25:20–24.
7. Skardal A, Mack D, Kapetanovic E, et al. Bioprinted amniotic fluid-derived stem cells accelerate healing of large skin wounds. Stem Cells Transl Med 2012;1:792–802.
8. Fisher C, Grahovac TL, Schafer ME, Shippert RD, Marra KG, Rubin JP. Comparison of harvest and processing techniques for fat grafting and adipose stem cell isolation. Plast Reconstr Surg 2013;132:351–361.
9. Nam Y, Rim YA, Lee J, Ju JH. Current therapeutic strategies for stem cell-based cartilage regeneration. Stem Cells Int 2018;2018:8490489.
10. Fabi SG, Goldman MP. Retrospective evaluation of micro-focused ultrasound for lifting and tightening the face and neck. Dermatol Surg 2014;40:569–575.
11. Jewell ML, Solish NJ, Desilets CS. Noninvasive body sculpting technologies with an emphasis on high-intensity focused ultrasound. Aesthet Plast Surg 2011;35:901–912.
12. Levin M. Bioelectric mechanisms in regeneration: Unique aspects and future perspectives. Semin Cell Dev Biol 2009;20:543–556.

13. Nevins M, Camelo M, Nevins ML, Schenk RK, Lynch SE. Periodontal regeneration in humans using recombinant human platelet-derived growth factor-BB (rhPDGF-BB) and allogenic bone. J Periodontol 2003;74:1282–1292.
14. Pegtel DM, Gould SJ. Exosomes. Ann Rev Biochem 2019;88:487–514.
15. Jing H, He X, Zheng J. Exosomes and regenerative medicine: State of the art and perspectives. Transl Res 2018;196:1–16.
16. Selmaj I, Mycko MP, Raine CS, Selmaj KW. The role of exosomes in CNS inflammation and their involvement in multiple sclerosis. J Neuroimmunol 2017;306:1–10.
17. Zavatti M, Beretti F, Casciaro F, Bertucci E, Maraldi T. Comparison of the therapeutic effect of amniotic fluid stem cells and their exosomes on monoiodoacetate-induced animal model of osteoarthritis. Biofactors 2020;46:106–117.

Chapter 12

What to Expect with Treatment

This chapter explains what to expect before, during, and after your treatments at CARE Esthetics. While these are minimally invasive treatments, certain guidelines must be followed. Most patients that elect to have treatments done at CARE Esthetics are seeking long-lasting regenerative outcomes. Below we present pretreatment and posttreatment instruction guidelines as well as general guidelines based on patient age.

General Guidelines By Age

Here we provide age-based guidelines for patients walking into our clinic for the very first time.

20s

By the time you turn 20, your skin begins to lose collagen at a rate of about 1.5% per year. Now is definitely a good time to start with quality skin care. Skin care regimens should include a cleanser (ideally something that is gentle on the skin), a regenerative agent that target the various skin layers effectively, and SPF sunscreen in the morning as well as something more regenerative at night.

Consider one or two natural regenerative therapies per year in your late 20s. These may include microneedling with PRF or laser peels. Because no volume loss is expected, no injections are needed, and many woman can maintain very good skin for years to come if they follow these regimens. If these simple measures are taken early, more aggressive treatments can be avoided later in life.

30s and 40s

Your skin will begin to show signs of aging. Now is the perfect time to start regenerative therapy. Provided no extensive sun damage is observed, we would typically recommend one Bio-CARE protocol per year. By investing in your skin now, you can save yourself from more extensive procedures down the line.

Continue to practice good skin care, and once it becomes more routine, you may venture into a more medical-grade cosmeceutical line. Remember that skin continues to lose collagen around 1.5% per year, but this is now compounding over previous decades. Ideally, you want to dramatically slow this down now, especially by the time you enter your 40s.

50s to 70s and beyond

When patients between the ages of 50 and 70 show up for the first time to our offices, visible signs of aging are already apparent. In such cases, a series of three Bio-CARE protocols are generally needed, approximately 1 month apart. This series will help kick-start those aging and "retired" fibroblast cells that bring collagen production back to full speed.

Depending on severity, typically two treatments are recommended on a yearly basis thereafter, one every 6 months, to refresh the skin and keep up collagen production for as long as desired.

Continue to use medical-grade skin care products. If you'd like more of a "booster," consider stronger retinols (higher concentration), but remember they are typically only utilized between therapies and only for a 3-month period. Otherwise they may cause increased irritation to the skin if used long-term.

What to Expect During a Bio-CARE Treatment

Pretreatment instructions

- Discontinue the use of Retin-A, retinols, vitamin A creams, and other topical medications 7 days before your microneedling treatment.

- Avoid alcohol, caffeine, and cigarettes for 3 days before and after your treatment. Smokers especially do not heal well due to lower blood flow, and more PRF will be needed to revascularize these tissues.
- For at least 3 days to 1 week prior to and after your treatment, avoid medicines or supplements that delay clotting such as aspirin, Motrin, ibuprofen, Aleve (all nonsteroidal anti-inflammatory agents), ginkgo biloba, garlic, flax oil, cod liver oil, vitamin A, vitamin E, or any other essential fatty acids. Remember: We are creating inflammation and need platelets to clot effectively. Use Tylenol if needed.
- Prescription medications (including heart and blood pressure medication) should be taken as prescribed right up to, and including, the day of and the day after your treatments.
- Avoid excessive sun or heat exposure at least 3 days prior to your appointment.
- Avoid tanning beds for at least 2 weeks prior to treatment.
- Avoid wearing ANY makeup on the day of your appointment. We will likely be microneedling, and we do not want to send makeup/chemicals into the skin.
- Increase your intake of fluids the day before your procedure by simply drinking two glasses of water in the morning, two glasses at lunch, and two glasses at dinner, in addition to your normal intake of water.
- Drink A LOT of water on the day of your appointment.
- Drink a full bottle of water (500 mL) at least 2 hours before your session.
- Avoid eating for 2 hours before your session.
- If you have a history of HSV infections (oral cold sores), you will be required to take antiviral medication (valacyclovir, acyclovir) for 2 days prior to treatment and 3 days after. Please notify the staff!

The most important thing to do before your procedure is to avoid vitamin A/retinols!

> Retinols are known to increase cell turnover by the removal of fine layers of skin (essentially acting like a very minor chemical peel conducted on a nightly basis). While this certainly helps prevent wrinkles when utilized long-term, always remember that it also will cause additional irritation, both during and after treatment. Therefore, please avoid retinols for 1 week before and after treatment!

During the procedure

For first-time CARE Esthetics patients, we take everything a bit slower to explain step by step all that goes into each procedure. We understand that this is new to you, and you might be nervous or have questions.

Regarding the laser, imagine having a warm flashlight that is fully controllable. For some individuals, we may need to turn up the intensity, yet for others we may need to turn it down. Some need longer bursts of energy, while others need shorter ones. The amazing thing about this technology is that we have full control over each of these parameters. The procedures should absolutely never be uncomfortable. The goal is to deliver as much laser energy as possible into the various treatment tissues, but never in a way that causes pain or significant discomfort. **Thus, we encourage you to give us as much feedback as possible!** This actually helps us design your customized treatment plan.

Typically, we will survey the face for things that may bother you. The odd dark spot (age/sun spot), maybe some veins around your nose or chin, or some unwanted facial hair. We can definitely address all of those! It is a good idea to survey your face prior to coming to our clinic and provide us with any and all feedback.

Expect that we won't treat everything all at once, despite our desire (and likely yours also) to maybe do so. This is by design.

Skin is a very reactive organ. We lean on the cautious side with all of our patients! Even if treatments are deemed 98% successful, we know you may just be in that 2%! As a result, if for instance you have many discolorations on your face caused by sun damage (age spots), we probably won't treat them all in the first session. First we will opt to treat a few age spots in less visible areas (maybe the side of the face or behind the ear) and observe in 1 week and 1 month how that tissue has healed.

At 1 week, we can observe and determine if the tissue reacted in a way that we expected. If you happen to be in that 2%, we might shift gears and focus on treating specifically your skin with a different treatment modality. This is the beauty of the CARE Esthetics model; collectively we've seen thousands and thousands of patients, so we are experts at what we do. If you are in that 2% group, we have established protocols where we can easily pivot and use a different laser setting to treat your age spot accordingly.

> We always err on the side of caution!

The end of the standard Bio-CARE protocol involves microneedling. A topical numbing cream is applied to remove discomfort, and the healing is very fast (24 hours) because we're able to get the PRF into and under the various skin layers. You'll be fully numb, but if you are uncomfortable, ask to have the depth of the microneedling device modified and/or if it is possible to reapply topical cream. The goal is for you to be entirely comfortable throughout the procedure.

After the treatment is completed, your skin will be pinkish. This is totally expected, especially if we are using PRF. Ideally you want to stay this way for 6 hours while the growth factors from your PRF soak into your skin. While this may seem alarming at first, the redness will be significantly decreased within 24 to 48 hours. Do not worry! It's part of the healing and regeneration process, and this protocol was specifically designed to treat you in a way that maximizes your results.

> Remember that we are using a product derived from your own concentrated blood, so YES, you will be red!

Posttreatment instructions

Things to do:
- Drink at least 64 ounces of water the day of treatment and each day for 1 week afterward. Hydration is key for good recovery and skin health.
- Do not touch, press, rub, or manipulate treated areas for at least 8 hours.
- Ice may be applied for 10 minutes on and 10 minutes off after the procedure for swelling/bruising in injected areas (if needed).
- No sunscreen OR makeup can be worn for 24 hours following treatment.
- Apply Aquaphor posttreatment as often as desired when skin dryness occurs. Aquaphor may be applied several times per day. After 24 hours, begin utilizing the Čuvget vitamin ampoules with PRF both morning and night.
- Wash the face MINIMALLY 6 hours after treatment. Use a gentle cleanser, such as Cetaphil. Gently massage the face with tepid water (a shower can provide an easier ability to massage the face while washing at the same time), and remove all serum and dried blood. This will improve the appearance of the skin and also allow for better subsequent product application, such as Čuvget.
- Keep the vitamin ampoules containing PRF in the refrigerator for maximum potency.

- After 48 to 72 hours following treatment, you can return to your regular skin care regimen with Čuvget products being applied both morning and evening.
- Minimal makeup can be applied after 72 hours posttreatment, but continue to use a gentle cleanser, Čuvget skin care products, and sunblock with an SPF of 25 or higher. If a more aggressive treatment was performed, use a more occlusive balm such as Aquaphor.
- Avoid alcohol-based toners for 7 days as well as excessive sun exposure for 10 days minimum. If red, stay out of the sun!
- For treatment of acne scars, usually three to five treatments are recommended, each 4 weeks apart.
- For scalp applications, shampoo and condition your scalp daily starting from the first evening or the next morning after PRF.

It is normal to experience possible bruising, redness, itching, soreness, and swelling, which usually subside within 24 to 48 hours but may last from 3 to 10 days following your procedure. Arnica and bromelain are helpful to decrease bruising and swelling.

Tylenol may be taken for discomfort/pain (very rare). Again, avoid NSAIDs such as Advil and aspirin.

What to avoid:
To ensure the proper healing environment, be certain to observe the following:

- For at least 1 month posttreatment, do NOT use any alpha hydroxy acids, beta hydroxy acid, retinol (vitamin A), vitamin C (in a low pH formula), or anything perceived as "active" skin care. You can use your Čuvget products as advised, as this is more of a regenerative skin care line.
- Avoid retinols in particular when sun spots are removed, as the redness following treatment will certainly persist in duration. Redness will eventually disappear, but this can be extended to several weeks/months if excessive skin products are used prior to complete healing. Avoid direct sunlight on such red spots while they are healing.
- Avoid intentional and direct sunlight, tanning beds, and heat exposure for 3 days.
- Do not go swimming for at least 24 hours posttreatment.

- Do not exercise or do strenuous activity for 2 days posttreatment. Sweating and gym environments are harmful, rife with bacteria, and may cause adverse reactions.
- If blistering or scabbing occurs, do not pick or remove scabs. This could lead to unintentional scarring. Wash your face twice daily with a gentle cleanser.

Other things to expect

Vascular lesions such as small facial varicose veins will lighten or change in color, often turning gray or bluish-purple. The lesions will typically lighten over the next week. Because the vessel has been ablated, the blood is slowly being removed, hence the color change, but this will fade over time.

If your skin remains red/discolored and you entered the clinic with rosacea as a precondition, your doctor may also prescribe hydroquinone. As reviewed in chapter 10, this can help resolve discolorations, and you may begin using it 1 month posttreatment.

If your skin begins to peel in random patterns (almost like a flaky sunburn), you probably aren't using the recommended exfoliating cleanser (we observe this most often in patients who don't follow that instruction). The Čuvget Exfoliating Cleanser in particular is effective after laser peels and is reasonably priced. At the minimum, use a gentle exfoliator to assist in the healing and desired treatment outcomes.

It is possible to have bruising or swelling after injections. That's normal for all fillers and is short-lived. If you do notice bruising, apply ice for 15 minutes every 1 to 2 hours. This will dramatically reduce the swelling and improve the healing.

You may experience itchy skin on the neck following laser treatment in particular. This is simply your lymphatic tissue at work—your body is draining your stored toxins from the skin. The itching goes away quickly and does not require any special treatment. You can apply ice to the area if it is uncomfortable, but it generally resolves within 24 to 48 hours.

We will want to see you 1 week after your procedure. Tell us EVERYTHING. By charting your healing and reactions to treatment, we will be able to further customize your therapy depending on the outcomes and downtime. Remember: The more tissue "damage" created, the better the results!

See you soon!